BREASTFEEDING
AND
NATURAL
CHILD SPACING

How Ecological Breastfeeding
Spaces Babies

by Sheila Matgen Kippley

Fourth Edition

The Couple to Couple League International, Inc.
Cincinnati, Ohio

Publisher
The Couple to Couple League International, Inc.
Location
4290 Delhi Pike
Cincinnati, OH 45238
Mailing address
P.O. Box 111184
Cincinnati, OH 45211
U.S.A.
E-mail
ccli@ccli.org
Website
www.ccli.org

First edition: K Publishers, 1969
Second edition: Harper and Row Publishers, Inc., New York, 1974
Paperback edition: Penguin Books, Inc. 1975
Third edition: Couple to Couple League International, Inc., 1989
Fourth edition: Couple to Couple League International, Inc., 1999

Cataloging data
L.C. 99-075775

Kippley, Sheila Matgen
Breastfeeding and Natural Child Spacing: How Ecological Breastfeeding Spaces Babies

1. Breastfeeding
2. Parenting
3. Natural family planning
4. Family planning
5. Birth control

Printing: 10   9   8   7   6   5   4   3   2

ISBN 0-926412-20-5

649.33

Acknowledgments

This book could not have been written in its present form without the help of others. Thus I want to thank all of the publishers who graciously gave me permission to quote from their publications. The many mothers who told me their experiences either personally or by mail made an invaluable contribution to the writing of this book. To each of them I express my deep thanks. Many readers will recognize that I have been influenced by La Leche League. I freely and gratefully acknowledge my great debt to that organization.

There are several individuals who have been of special help in preparing the fourth edition. John DuMont of the Couple to Couple League Headquarters arranged the photo shoot and helped with the cover design. My daughter Margaret previously appeared as the four-year-old in the title page illustration, and now she's on the cover with her own child. My thanks to her and her husband for the cover photo. Also at the CCL Headquarters, Virginia Niehaus did her usual fine job of proofreading, and Keith Bower used his wonderful computer skills to lay out the text. Publications Editor Ann Gundlach deserves a special thanks not only for her expertise in cover design and shepherding the text from my word processor to publication, but also for her patience. Certainly she must have thought more than once, "How many changes can there be?" but she never complained. Lastly, my husband has been my chief editor. His hours reviewing the manuscript have improved this book greatly, and I am grateful for his input and suggestions.

Table of Contents

Foreword

For many years the value of breastfeeding has been recognized, especially in terms of the close bond it establishes between a mother and her child and the health benefits of a natural form of nourishing infants. It is therefore heartening to see a revived interest in this natural form of nurturing. However, there is another dimension of breastfeeding that is not as widely known, that is, choosing breastfeeding as a natural means for spacing births.

Used in this way, breastfeeding has been found to be of particular value, not only in various traditional cultures, where such an approach has been known for centuries, but in the wider world. As one of the natural ways for regulating fertility, breastfeeding thus takes its place among various methods that constitute the "authentic alternative" to contraception, and so it remains a subject for research and study.

When, in the light of *serious reasons*, a husband and wife decide to postpone the birth of their next child, they must nevertheless remain open to God's gift of new life. Therefore, in making the next decision about the *method* of spacing births, they will draw on what the Creator has provided within the body of a woman. They will respect God's plan for life and love and say "yes" to the Lord of Life. As Pope John Paul II teaches... they are acting as "ministers" of God's plan (cf. *Familiaris Consortio*, 32).

As they serve the divine plan and cooperate with the Creator, the natural benefits of the cycles and processes that God provides are soon evident. These benefits are particularly obvious in the nurturing and nourishing of breastfeeding. Here we have a tangible example of the positive value of the natural way of transmitting human life.

I am sure that those who study *Breastfeeding and Natural Child Spacing* will be grateful to Sheila Kippley for her continuing work of explaining and promoting this natural way that offers so much to families.

Alfonso Cardinal López Trujillo
President of the Pontifical Council for the Family

Introduction

This manual is a book of its times. Several hundred years ago it would have been superfluous because breastfeeding was the general practice, and 100 years ago it would have been impossible because of the lack of research at that time. Today, however, I think this book fills a need.

This book initially grew out of a great many conversations I had with other mothers who shared with me a common interest in providing our babies with the benefits of breastfeeding and in having the side effect of natural child spacing. All of us ran up against what seemed to be a nearly universal skepticism about both of these common interests — at least at the level of homemaker hearsay. On the other hand, at the level of medical research, our common interests were bolstered. When I frequently found myself playing the role of transmitter of scientific information about breastfeeding and child spacing, I decided that there was a general knowledge gap on the part of many mothers and doctors that might be narrowed by a book of this type.

More important, the methods advocated in this manual provided a double service to friends of mine who had previously been unsuccessful in their earlier attempts at breastfeeding. First of all, they became successful as nursing mothers and, as a result, came to a greater enjoyment of their babies. Secondly, they experienced a form of child spacing for which they were not only grateful but which some of them had believed could not be achieved through nursing.

The particular information that all of us needed clarified was the possibility of becoming pregnant while nursing. I came to realize that some mothers were weaning very early for fear of early postpartum pregnancy even though they sincerely wanted to breastfeed their babies. Some of these fears were real because of cultural interference with natural breastfeeding; almost all were the result of inadequate information. I found that a review of the medical research in this area, plus the adoption of the ecological breastfeeding program described in this manual, gave mothers confidence, peace of mind, and the enjoyment of continued nursing.

I want to stress at the outset that breastfeeding is far more than a merely biological function. It is frequently an emotional experience for both mother and baby; it is truly interpersonal. You as a breastfeeding mother are not just fulfilling a mammary function, but you are also contributing to the personal fulfillment of yourself as a mother and to the emotional security and development of your baby. This type of natural mothering can be very rewarding.

This is not a book on birth control as such, although I fully realize that some may be interested in what is written here primarily from the point of view of finding an efficient means of child spacing that meets the moral criteria of everyone. It is not within the scope of this book to delve deeply into a discussion of moral principles. Rather, my purpose here is to show that for whatever reason breastfeeding is used, it can be an effective means of spacing children. I will say, however, that the more you think in terms of doing what is most in accord with nature and what is best for your baby, the more easily you will be able to carry out the program outlined here. Furthermore, it is somewhat doubtful whether you would be able to sustain the criticism you might get from well-meaning friends and advisers if you looked at breastfeeding only as a means of birth control. And one doesn't become a member of the smart set by extended breastfeeding although some extremely smart women are doing it. Breastfeeding entails a loving personal relationship between mother and baby, and I wonder if the mother who looked upon her suckling baby primarily as a birth-control device would be able to maintain that nursing relationship of love for very long. A baby can sense his mother's attitude toward him from the way in which she nurses him, and no one would want to see such a naturally loving relationship distorted. For the mother who may start out with a poor attitude toward her child, however, I think that with a little bit of self-giving there is a much greater chance of her growing to accept, love, and appreciate her baby through breastfeeding than through the use of such artifacts as bottles, formulas, messy baby foods, and pacifiers.

I have been encouraged by endorsements of extended breastfeeding by health organizations and a world religious leader. The American Academy of Pediatrics promotes exclusive breastfeeding for the first six months of life and asks mothers to nurse their babies for at least one year. UNICEF and the WHO also promote exclusive breastfeeding for the first six months of life and ask mothers to nurse their babies up to the second year of life or beyond. In 1995 Pope John Paul II addressed a scientific conference on breastfeeding. He endorsed the UNICEF recommendations and also encouraged mothers to breastfeed up to the second year of life or beyond.

A word about pronouns. I refer to the baby as masculine. Many sentences and paragraphs talk about both the mother and baby, and it is much easier to keep the pronouns straight by referring to the baby as he, him, and his.

I hope that no one will take offense at my efforts to paraphrase the Man from Nazareth. Speaking of the relationship of secular values and the kingdom of God, He said, "Seek first the kingdom of God and all these other things will be given unto you." What I have been trying to say is that, by seeking first to do what is in accord with God's natural plan, other benefits will follow.

This fourth edition has undergone many small changes throughout the book to bring it up to date. The primary additions are the inclusion and emphasis of "The Seven Standards" for breastfeeding infertility, especially during the first six months postpartum, and the chapter devoted to "The Crucial First Three Years."

In summary, this book is published so that mothers will come to enjoy the same satisfying relationship with their babies that I have experienced. I hope that they will also, if that is what they want, come to enjoy the derivative effect of natural child spacing. At the least, they and whoever else is interested will learn about some of the research that has been done concerning breastfeeding and natural infertility, why the Seven Standards are important for natural infertility during the first six months postpartum, what is meant by ecological breastfeeding, its many advantages for the individual baby and mother, and its normal effect of child spacing.

Sheila Matgen Kippley

1

Breastfeeding *Does* Space Babies

Ecological breastfeeding

Natural child spacing is very easy to teach. It is also easy to do when the mother remains with her baby or keeps the baby close to her side. There are three mothering behaviors that are common when a mother follows the ecological breastfeeding program and experiences natural child spacing. These are listed below.

- A mother is physically close to her baby; frequently she holds and carries him.
- She nurses and pacifies her baby frequently at the breast.
- She lies down and nurses her baby during a nap and during the night.

This form of natural mothering is often referred to as "ecological breastfeeding," and this is a good place to explain the meaning of that phrase. Strictly speaking, ecology is concerned with the relationship between living things and their environment. Frequently it is a rather delicate relationship, and every year we read about how this or that animal or fish or tree may be affected by a change in the environment. The language of ecology is applied less frequently to human relationships, but it is still valid. For example, there is a gentle, ecological relationship between the breastfeeding baby and his mother. The more the baby nurses, the more milk she has for him.

Another aspect of this breastfeeding ecology is the relationship between the emotional and physiological needs of the infant. Both needs are satisfied at the breast. The hungry baby gets not only nutrition but also emotional satisfaction at the breast and through being picked up and held. The baby who nurses primarily for emotional satisfaction also gets some nourishment, and simultaneously he helps reinforce his mother's milk supply. The mother can continue to satisfy the emotional need at the breast even when her baby has a nutritional need for other foods in addition to breastmilk. This helps to explain why some cultures that are sensitive to the child's needs think nothing of continuing breastfeeding for three or more years.

Breastfeeding plays an important role in the emotional development of the mother as well. For this reason breastfeeding is not only the best start for the baby, but it is also the best start for the mother. The nursing relationship gives her a feeling of self-importance and self-worth as a mother from

1

the satisfaction gained in meeting her baby's needs herself. Breastfeeding provides a natural and easy way for the mother to learn how to be a good mother and to gain confidence in her mothering abilities. The rewards in giving, especially to one's small children, are emotional ones that cannot be measured.

Last but not least, the frequent stimulation of the breast by the baby plays an extremely important role in maintaining natural infertility after childbirth. Frequent and unrestricted suckling is the most important factor in maintaining breastfeeding infertility. Such frequency is brought about by satisfying your baby's needs — both nutritional and emotional — at your breast. This and other aspects of the breastfeeding ecology will be spelled out in later chapters. Suffice it to say that Mother Nature has provided a mutually beneficial relationship in breastfeeding.

Natural child spacing

The rules for breastfeeding and natural child spacing can be very specific. They are few and can be written on a small index card. We now call these rules the **Seven Standards** of ecological breastfeeding.

1. Do exclusive breastfeeding for the first six months of life; don't use other liquids and solids.

2. Pacify your baby at your breasts.

3. Don't use bottles and pacifiers. (You provide the best nourishment and pacification for your baby.)

4. Sleep with your baby for night feedings. (Once you get accustomed to it, you will love lying-down nursing.)

5. Sleep with your baby for a daily-nap feeding. (You need the nap almost as much as he does.)

6. Nurse frequently day and night, and avoid schedules.

7. Avoid any practice that restricts nursing or separates you from your baby.

In addition, wean your baby gradually at his pace. Today many authorities are encouraging mothers to nurse for at least two years.

The above rules describe the type of nursing we call ecological breastfeeding. Notice that two of the rules mean you actually nurse your baby during your sleep. With experience you can learn to do this. Isn't it interesting that God has provided a plan for mother and baby in which breastfeeding infertility becomes more effective when the mother is sleeping and also nursing her baby?

The heart and core of ecological breastfeeding is frequent and unrestricted nursing, and the key behavior of natural child spacing is mother/baby togetherness. Obviously you must be available to your baby to meet his needs and to care for him. When you are available to your baby, the frequent and unrestricted nursing required for natural child spacing happens automatically. To repeat, ecological breastfeeding is easy to do when you remain physically close to your baby.

Through breastfeeding alone, babies can be spaced 18 to 30 months apart. If mothers follow the ecological breastfeeding program in this book, they will experience 14 months of amenorrhea after childbirth, on the average. Amenorrhea means the absence of menstruation — no periods. In fact, the nine months of infertility that a woman experiences during pregnancy usually continues for another 9, 14, 20 or more months through breastfeeding. The baby has merely switched positions.

Unknown to many is the fact that ecological breastfeeding is the most effective method of family planning during the first six months postpartum provided that the mother remains in amenorrhea and is following the Seven Standards. The chance of a mother conceiving during the first three months postpartum while doing ecological breastfeeding and remaining in amenorrhea is almost nil. The chance of her conceiving during the next three months postpartum while doing ecological breastfeeding and remaining in amenorrhea is 1%. Or in other words, during the first six months postpartum, ecological breastfeeding provides the nursing mother in amenorrhea a totally natural 99% rate of infertility!

Breastfeeding infertility is the result of a purely biological act, the act of breastfeeding. This natural method excludes all unnatural forms of birth control. It has nothing to do with abstinence. Breastfeeding infertility is achieved by the constant mothering that occurs at the woman's breasts. That's why this type of breastfeeding is also called natural mothering.

When a woman nurses her baby as nature intended she will notice an absence of menstruation. Her ovaries remain at rest. There is no cyclic activity. It is true that eventually menstruation will return while the mother is nursing. However menstruation was not meant to occur within three months after childbirth. Women were meant to have a lengthy absence of menstruation due to breastfeeding; their cyclic activity was intended by nature to return at a much later date. To repeat, it is perfectly normal for a nursing mother to go nine months, one year, two years or more without any menstruation.

In the following chapters I give more detailed information and support for this natural method of child spacing. I believe that many parents will adopt the ecological breastfeeding program because of their primary interest in breastfeeding infertility. Eventually parents who become involved in this type of mothering and fathering will learn the many other benefits of breastfeeding for themselves, their children and for their family. For couples who want to space their children only through breastfeeding, this book will offer you the necessary information and support.

For those desiring a quick overview of the ecological breastfeeding program associated with natural child spacing, a summary follows.

Summary of Ecological Breastfeeding and Natural Child Spacing Program

Basic principles

1. Frequent and unrestricted nursing is the primary factor in producing natural lactation amenorrhea and infertility. (Lactation amenorrhea is the absence of menstruation due to breastfeeding.)

2. Ecological breastfeeding almost always provides this frequent nursing and natural infertility. It is that type of baby care which follows the natural mother-baby relationship. It avoids the use of artifacts and mother substitutes; it follows the baby-initiated patterns. Ecological breastfeeding is the norm and offers many built-in benefits, one of which is extended natural infertility. In essence, a lengthy postpartum amenorrhea is the expected norm.

Phase I of ecological breastfeeding: The Seven Standards

This phase almost invariably produces natural infertility as long as the program is complete. Phase I usually lasts six months. The key to natural infertility is frequent and unrestricted nursing. The following Seven Standards help to ensure this frequent nursing.

1. Do exclusive breastfeeding for the first six months of life; don't use other liquids and solids.
2. Pacify your baby at your breasts.
3. Don't use bottles and pacifiers.
4. Sleep with your baby for night feedings.
5. Sleep with your baby for a daily-nap feeding.
6. Nurse frequently day and night, and avoid schedules.
7. Avoid any practice that restricts nursing or separates you from your baby.

Phase II of ecological breastfeeding: The Six Standards

• Phase II of ecological breastfeeding begins when your baby starts taking solids or liquids other than breastmilk.

• You begin to give liquids when your baby shows an interest in the cup, usually after six months.

• Aside from Standard #1, exclusive breastfeeding, the other Six Standards of Phase I will remain operative until the baby gradually loses interest in breastfeeding. Phase II is a very gradual program in which the amount of nursing is 1) not decreased at all at first, and 2) lessened only gradually at baby's pace. Phase II is frequently longer than Phase I with regard to natural infertility if ecological breastfeeding continues with frequent and unrestricted nursing.

Return of fertility

The First 6 Months. The *first 8 weeks postpartum* for the exclusively breastfeeding mother are so infertile that in 1988 scientists agreed that any vaginal bleeding during the first 56 days postpartum can be ignored for determining amenorrhea or fertility for the exclusively breastfeeding mother. This rule would apply also to the ecological breastfeeding mother.

During the *first 3 months postpartum*, the chance of pregnancy occurring is practically nil if the ecological breastfeeding mother remains in amenorrhea.

During the *next 3 months postpartum*, there is only a 1% chance of pregnancy if the ecological breastfeeding mother continues to remain in amenorrhea.

After 6 Months. For the nursing mother there is about a 6% chance of pregnancy occurring prior to the first menstruation. This assumes no fertility awareness and unrestricted intercourse. This risk can be reduced to close to 1% through the techniques of systematic natural family planning — observing the signs of fertility and abstaining accordingly.

About 70% of ecological breastfeeding mothers experience their first menstruation between 9 and 20 months postpartum. The average return of menstruation for ecological breastfeeding mothers is between 14 and 15 months.

Natural spacing by breastfeeding alone

For those couples who desire 18 to 30 months between the births of their children, ecological breastfeeding should be sufficient.

Support needed

With small print, this chapter could be printed on two sides of one sheet of paper, so why do we have a whole book? In a bottlefeeding, early weaning culture, you need intellectual and emotional support to do ecological breastfeeding. I think you will find it in the chapters that follow.

Your Baby's Sucking Needs

The breast for nourishment

One of a baby's strongest needs is the need to suck — and rightly so, for it's his primary means of obtaining nourishment in the early weeks and months after birth. The nursing of an infant stimulates the production of milk in his mother and is the natural means of transmitting milk from mother to baby.

Lactation, or the production of milk in the mother's body, is influenced proportionately by the amount of stimulation the breast receives. This stimulation is most frequently caused by the nursing of the infant. (A weaker stimulation is the expression of milk by hand or pump.) The more stimulation the breast receives, the more milk it will supply or produce. The exact opposite is likewise true. When a baby weans himself gradually from the breast or is weaned by his mother who introduces foods or formula so that her baby requires less from the breast, then her supply of milk is lessened accordingly. Lactation is a delicate process, for the supply of milk almost always meets the demands, whether that demand is great or small.

The following story illustrates how a mother's milk supply is influenced largely by her baby's demand at the breast. A friend introduced solids early at the advice of her doctor. Unlike her previous doctor, this new doctor insisted on solids at six weeks even though he strongly approved of breast-feeding. As soon as she followed his instructions, her milk supply decreased, she became depressed, and menstruation returned. Several months later a letter came, telling me that her supply had increased:

> "Of course, I'm still nursing Jeff. He only has solids once a day. Frank and I both felt we should cut down on the solids, and we had a good chance to do so over the Easter holidays when we traveled to Salt Lake. He had very little extra, and I feel this brought back or brought on more milk. Makes me happier."

It is amazing to learn how effective the demand for milk can be in producing the supply. There are mothers who start supplementary bottlefeedings and then want to eliminate them. By doubling or tripling the number of nursings at the breast for one or two days, the mother will usually have plenty of milk and can discontinue the bottlefeeding.

Another example is the mother who delivers a premature or sick baby. She may express her milk regularly to maintain a supply until her baby comes home. Over a period of six weeks one mother expressed her milk into a sterile jar that she took daily to the hospital to nourish her premature, incubator baby. Her supply increased from 1½ ounces to over 20 ounces per day during this period. She met up with much resistance at first, and everyone thought it wasn't possible. At a later date the pediatrician told her to wean the baby to a bottle by six months of age, saying that the nursing wouldn't do her or the baby any good. Being well read on the subject of breastfeeding, she ignored this advice, and both she and the baby prospered.

A few mothers have produced some milk for the baby they planned to adopt. One mother wrote that she was actually producing milk prior to adoption. In another case the adopting mother had not recently given birth; she was without any supply of milk and she was without the normal hormonal and physiological changes of late pregnancy that provide an adequate and easy milk supply after childbirth. She was, so to speak, bone dry; yet she persevered and developed a milk supply for her adopted baby.

Needless to say, such a process isn't recommended to just anybody, for it takes a considerable amount of constant effort and a very strong desire to nurse one's baby. In addition, it takes a baby who is agreeable to the idea, for by the time an adoptive mother receives her baby, the infant may have been bottlefed for several weeks. It takes more work to get milk from the breast than from the bottle, and some babies are not particularly disposed toward making the transition.

Nature also provides an ample supply of milk to those mothers who have twins. One doctor insisted that his patient nurse her twin babies because he felt it would be easier for her. I have a friend who had two sets of twins and found this to be true. It is the only way a mother can feed two babies at the same time.

In addition, a few mothers with one breast have been encouraged by their doctors to nurse in order to reduce the chance of developing cancer in the remaining breast. The American Cancer Society and the National Cancer Institute report that cancer of the breast is more apt to develop in those breasts that do not give milk, and scientific studies confirm the fact that long-term nursing lowers the breast cancer risk.

These examples are given to show not only how lactation can occur under unusual or different circumstances but above all to impress upon you, as a mother, that you certainly can nurse your baby under normal conditions. The important thing to remember is that breastfeeding can be a very easy and natural affair. God gave you your baby and He also provided you with the best food for your baby, food that you alone can give him. To help you feed your baby, He gave your infant a strong urge to suck. It's that simple. Let the baby nurse often at the breast, and you will have plenty of milk for nourishment.

The breast for pacification

This brings us to another important point. Babies have an obvious need to comfort nurse. They will mouth anything they come in contact with — breast, fingers, clothing, or objects. This is a normal, healthy habit that should be encouraged. The baby or older child will outgrow this need easily later if his desire to nurse for comfort as well as nourishment isn't frustrated early in life. It's a need that is particularly well satisfied at his mother's breast.

The breast is nature's pacifier for the baby. This is hard for many mothers to appreciate in our culture where bottlefeeding is the preferred method of feeding and where breastfeeding mothers are encouraged to use a bottle when a feeding takes place outside the home. We tend to ignore the fact that these artificial aids — bottles and pacifiers — are merely substitutes for the mother or her breast. The infant's need to be pacified at the breast is nature's way of bringing mother and baby together at other than feeding times. The breast can have a very calming effect upon the baby. This is why it is so easy to nurse a baby to sleep. The breastfed baby wants the breast for this "pacifying" need of his just as a bottlefed baby prefers his bottle or soother. This is why the nursing mother cannot really say how many times she has fed her baby during the day. Does she count the times she has pacified her baby into a deep sleep — even though her baby might have acquired little milk in the process? The breast, besides offering security and comfort, brings love and reassurance any time during the day or night.

Suckling is apparently a very satisfying experience for infants. Dr. James Hymes, author of *The Child Under Six*,[1] says that suckling provides babies with many pleasant sensations, and in *The First Nine Months*[2] Geraldine Lux Flanagan points out that some babies are born with a callus on their thumbs as a result of their sucking activity in the womb. Surely this is an indication that sucking was a satisfying experience for these babies even before birth.

Sucking stimulation and ovulation

When a young girl reaches puberty, she normally begins to experience the menstrual cycle. If she has prepared for this as a natural development, she accepts it as part of becoming an adult woman and may give it little further thought. On the other hand, if she wanted a better understanding of her bodily functions, she may have sought out the whole story behind her monthly cycle. If you are such a woman, the following facts will scarcely be new; but certain facts take on new relevance when seen in relation to childbearing and child spacing.

A baby girl at birth has two ovaries which contain all the eggs (or ova) that she will ever have. At puberty her ovaries become active, and during each fertility-menstrual cycle an egg develops and approaches the surface of the ovary. When its individual container, called a follicle, ruptures, the egg or ovum is released from the ovary and is now free to travel from the ovary through the Fallopian tube toward the womb or uterus. The release of an ovum is called ovulation and is necessary before fertilization or conception can take place.

While your body is preparing for ovulation, the lining of your uterus is thickening to receive the newly conceived human life should conception occur. If the ovum is not fertilized, the lining of the uterus is sloughed off and bleeding occurs. This bleeding is known as menstruation, and it's often referred to as a "menstrual period."

If pregnancy occurs, however, a change occurs in the body chemistry. One effect of this is that the lining of the womb is not sloughed off but remains built up, thereby eliminating menstrual bleeding during pregnancy. This is termed pregnancy amenorrhea. Another effect of this change in the body chemistry during pregnancy is that the ovaries remain at rest; no additional ovulations and pregnancies can occur until after childbirth. The only exception would be multiple conceptions, but when double or triple ovulations occur in a cycle, they all occur within the same 24-hour period.

Our interest in this whole process is the continuation of this infertile condition following childbirth. If the mother nurses her baby properly, she will normally retain this infertile condition by experiencing a lengthy absence from menstrual periods following childbirth. This is called lactation amenorrhea. Medical researchers have been unable to describe with certainty the body chemistry involved, but there is widespread agreement that the amount of nursing by the infant at the breast is the most important factor in providing this natural infertility.

To maintain breastfeeding amenorrhea, two types of nursing are needed: 1) frequent nursing and 2) unrestricted or uninterrupted nursing. Frequent nursing usually occurs when mother and baby are alert during the day. Unrestricted nursing usually occurs when mother and baby are sleeping together for mother's daily nap or during the night. While the mother is sleeping, the baby can nurse to his heart's content without any interruption.

Breastfeeding stimulates hormones to respond within the mother's body, and these hormones respond in surges. Nursing has to be frequent in order to produce enough of those surges to keep the mother in amenorrhea. Most mothers need lots of stimulation in order to remain in deep amenorrhea following childbirth. Frequent and unrestricted nursings experienced day and night by the mother usually provide this ample stimulation.

There are two practical conclusions for the nursing mother who would like the side benefit of breastfeeding infertility. First of all, she should positively cooperate with her baby's natural desires to nurse whether it be for nutritional or emotional needs. Second, she should avoid those practices that prematurely reduce her baby's feeding at the breast. This would include almost the entire range of cultural baby care practices in the United States: early solids and liquids other than mother's milk, rigid nursing schedules, pacifiers, the race to get baby sleeping through the night, babysitters, and so on.

The guidelines that are given in this book go hand in hand with what I call "natural mothering." By natural mothering I mean that care of an infant in which his needs are met primarily by his mother and not by artifacts or babysitters. It is natural baby care as well, for the mother follows her baby's natural development or pattern. Natural mothering, then, is not ruled by clocks or schedules; instead, the baby is the mother's guide.

[1] James Hymes, *The Child Under Six*, Englewood Cliffs: Prentice Hall, 1963.
[2] Geraldine Lux Flanagan, *The First Nine Months*, New York: Pocket Books, 1962.

3

Exclusive Breastfeeding

STANDARD ONE:
Do exclusive breastfeeding during the first six months of life.
Don't use other liquids and solids.

Nothing but mother's milk

The infertility of pregnancy has been compared with the infertility of breastfeeding, and the absence of ovulation and menstruation was noted in both. It's obvious that the baby developing in his mother's womb gets 100% of his nourishment from his mother. The point that cannot be overemphasized with regard to breastfeeding and ovulation is that the baby who gives his mother the natural infertility of breastfeeding will also be getting 100% of his nourishment from his mother's breasts, at least during the first six months of life. Less than 100% is weaning, and never do I want to give the impression that breastfeeding plus supplements during the early months provides the same degree of infertility that exclusive breastfeeding does.

Weaning actually begins when the mother introduces other foods or fluids to a breastfed baby. The weaning process can last two days, two weeks, twelve months, or three years or more. It begins as soon as the mother offers her baby nourishment other than breastmilk; it ends the day that her baby no longer takes any milk from the breast. From this definition it can be said that many mothers wean their babies from the day they leave the hospital, even though they may nurse for six months or longer. In addition, the baby also undergoes an emotional weaning from the breast, gradually receiving this emotional nourishment in other ways from his mother and from other sources and contacts.

In our society we are conditioned to look to physicians for help in every phase of life. Thus, it is sometimes difficult to be understood when speaking about exclusive breastfeeding. In the past, many doctors have prescribed formulas and have set up definite schedules for the introduction of juices, cereals, and solids — and some still do. The result is that many parents regard bottlefeeding as the norm and look upon breastfeeding as a nice but very short-run supplement to the "real" nourishment put out by the food and formula companies. Such parents are not well informed.

As the American Academy of Pediatrics now states, the early feeding of solids does *not* have a *rational* basis in health care except in very rare circumstances.[1] Parents, however, hope solid foods will help their babies go longer between feedings and help them sleep through the night. Other reasons given for early solids are 1) advertisements in lay and professional magazines, 2) the insistence of mothers or of doctors, and 3) the easy availability of baby cereals and pureed foods, and 4) the heavy use of formula and bottles.

Exclusive breastfeeding means that the baby derives all his food and liquid from his mother's breast. It means that the only nipples that need to be in the house are part of his mother's natural equipment. You do not need a single artificial nipple in the house. We raised our last four children without using bottles or pacifiers. With natural mothering and parenting, we did not need or miss them. (We didn't know better with our first.)

In December 1997, the American Academy of Pediatrics (AAP) issued a strong policy statement on breastfeeding.[2] The AAP endorsed exclusive breastfeeding for the first six months of life, stating that breastfeeding alone is not only sufficient but also best for the infant's health. The AAP specifically stated that no water, no other fluids or solids, and no fluoride should be given the baby during the first six months of life. The AAP also discouraged pacifiers for newborns.

Cultural nursing

When a nursing mother also uses bottles and pacifiers or other substitutes for her mothering or her milk, we call this cultural nursing. Cultural nursing is the type of nursing we often see in Westernized societies. The mother nurses, but she also offers other liquids via the bottle or she starts solids early. Pacifiers are used frequently. Strict schedules with regard to feeding or sleeping are common. Mother/baby separation occurs because babies are cared for by others.

With our first baby, I was interested in breastfeeding infertility, but my obstetrician warned me that I would have a period by three months postpartum no matter how I nursed. I did cultural nursing and had my first period by three months postpartum. Thankfully I had a different doctor with our next baby and began to learn the truth of the matter.

Exclusive breastfeeding not sufficient by itself

My second obstetrician knew I wanted to breastfeed and that I wanted some natural spacing. He said I must exclusively breastfeed, that I was to offer my baby only my milk. She was born during the hot summer months, so I asked about giving her water. He said "not even water." His advice to me was to call him as soon as I had my first menstrual period. Menstruation returned at one year postpartum. At that time we desired another baby and I never did make that phone call. We soon moved to another country, but I am forever grateful to this doctor.

I appreciate the fact that he did not tell me to exclusively breastfeed for only six months. This is the advice given today to mothers in different countries. If I had been told that breastfeeding could postpone fertility for only six months, I would not have written this book.

New studies support the infertility effectiveness of exclusive breast-feeding and amenorrhea during the first six months of life. For years La Leche League International, an international breastfeeding organization, taught that if you were exclusively breastfeeding and in amenorrhea, breastfeed-ing provided a 99% effectiveness rate during the first six months. This was confirmed in 1988 at a meeting in Bellagio, Italy where international ex-perts met to review the recent research on breastfeeding infertility. These experts came up with a consensus very similar to La Leche League's. They concluded that if a mother was "fully or nearly fully" breastfeeding and if she remained in amenorrhea (any vaginal bleeding up to the 56th day post-partum can be ignored), breastfeeding offered a 98% effectiveness rate dur-ing the first six months postpartum.[3] Today this "method" is called the Lac-tational Amenorrhea Method. The Bellagio Consensus stimulated further research to test the Lactational Amenorrhea Method, and such research has confirmed the effectiveness of this method.

My concern with the exclusive breastfeeding rule is that by itself exclu-sive breastfeeding does not maintain amenorrhea for many women during the first six months postpartum. Studies show that only 56% of exclusively breastfeeding mothers are maintaining amenorrhea during the entire six months postpartum.[4] On the other hand, 93% of those involved with eco-logical breastfeeding will remain in amenorrhea for the entire six months postpartum. The research on ecological breastfeeding is described more fully in Chapter 21.

One of the reasons that I maintained amenorrhea for six months post-partum while exclusively breastfeeding was due to the fact that I began to adopt other more natural childcare practices such as sleeping with the baby for a nap and during the night and not using a pacifier. For years, I have stressed that exclusive breastfeeding by itself is not sufficient to maintain amenorrhea or breastfeeding infertility. There are just too many women who experience an early return of menstruation at three or four months postpartum using the exclusive breastfeeding rule.

The truth of the matter is that when a mother provides 1) all of her baby's nourishment at her breast and 2) the greater part of his other sucking needs at her breast, she will almost invariably experi-ence the side effect of natural infertility. You can have natural child spacing (using systematic natural family planning) without breastfeeding, but you cannot normally have breastfeeding in the sense described above without the side effect of child spacing. To put it another way, if a woman should sincerely want to become pregnant within the first six months fol-lowing childbirth, she should not follow the breastfeeding plan described in this chapter and book.

15

I want to call special attention to the second part of the preceding statement in boldface type, "the greater part of his other sucking needs." Some mothers have been very disappointed to experience menstruation or conception while exclusively breastfeeding. Too often, however, these mothers are restricting the nursing by not following the other aspects of natural mothering. In other words, the exclusive breastfeeding rule is no guarantee that menstruation or ovulation will not occur. A mother who follows the exclusive breastfeeding *nutrition* rule may not be satisfying her child's other suckling needs at the breast. May I give you a true story?

A breastfeeding mother phoned for information on natural family planning — information that neither the hospital nor her doctor could give her. Knowing that she had nursed her babies, we discussed natural spacing. She wasn't initially interested in reading the material I had gathered on the subject, but I encouraged her to do so to see if she really was an exception — for she was convinced that she was the odd case. She had exclusively breastfed all her babies, yet experienced regular menstrual periods 3½ to 4 weeks after childbirth with all six children. She never once experienced an absence of periods while nursing. In addition, she was nursing her sixth baby often, day and night. Upon returning the material, she wrote:

> First an apology — someone had told me you were "far-out" and I accepted the opinion without investigation. Our problem in nursing probably lies in not letting Jane suck long enough. I usually have a fast flow. She is satisfied in about 8 to 10 minutes. I also have used both breasts to fill her up to save time. She sucks her finger, and this indicates a need for more sucking. I do nurse lying down as often as possible, but I've seldom let the baby fall asleep with me. I feel that my practice of nursing quickly also is at fault. Don't you? Let me try some of your suggestions and we'll see what happens.

The suggestions the mother was referring to were those in the material I had given her, as normally I do not suggest a change in nursing or mothering habits for those interested in natural family planning if menstruation has already occurred.

About six months later I happened to meet this mother and learned from her that she experienced lactation amenorrhea for the first time. Her baby was four months old when her periods stopped, and then she went four months without menstrual bleeding. This particular case illustrates that there is much more to natural spacing than merely filling baby's tummy or satisfying hunger pangs by exclusive breastfeeding.

In the past the exclusive breastfeeding nutrition rule was the only guideline taught to mothers who were interested in nursing and in avoiding an immediate pregnancy. True, that rule is extremely important, but it is only one aspect of the overall natural spacing picture. For breastfeeding infertility, other rules are also important and they deserve as much attention and emphasis.

[1] *Pediatrics*, December 1997, 1035-39.

[2] Ibid.

[3] "Consensus Statement: Breastfeeding as a Family Planning Method," *The Lancet*, November 19, 1988.

[4] Perez, A. and Valdes, V., "Santiago Breastfeeding Promotion Program: Preliminary Results of an Intervention Study," *Am. J. of Obst. Gyn.*, December 1991, 2039-40.

Pacification of the Baby

STANDARD TWO:
Pacify your baby at your breasts.

STANDARD THREE:
Don't use bottles and pacifiers.

The second standard

Pacifiers strongly influence mothering today. They are of special interest here since they limit the amount of nursing and mothering at the breast. In fact, when regularly offered, the pacifier often receives more attention from the baby than the bottle or the breast.

We have already noted the role that the breast plays in pacifying the baby. It is also true that not only the breast but the mother's entire body plays an important role here as well. Her body is very adaptable. Her fingers can stroke and tease. Her knuckle or chin can act as a "pacifier" when the baby does not desire the breast. Her face and voice offer expressions of love and happiness that tell the baby that he is someone very special. Her body offers motion and rhythm — two things babies love and which they receive when their mothers hold them, rock them, or carry them. The mother provides an "infant seat" for her baby when she sits and crosses one knee. Certain leg positions can form a cradle for her baby; when her legs move, baby is gently rocked. Babies need a good mother, and no one can replace her. Sometimes her presence is all that is needed to change a baby's cries into smiles. Truly, a mother is the best pacifier for her baby.

Why a pacifier?

The most obvious reason for offering the pacifier is to soothe and comfort the baby. Today many parents encourage the use of the pacifier almost permanently so that their baby is usually seen with a pacifier glued to his mouth or pinned to his clothing. Indirectly the pacifier also pacifies the parent who is thus spared the trouble of nursing or holding the baby. Some nursing mothers claim that they can't get along without the pacifier. Their babies are too fussy, the mothers have too much milk, or the parents are concerned about thumbsucking. Let's take a look at these reasons.

"The baby is too fussy"

It can be expected that most babies will have an occasional fussy spell. This doesn't mean that it will happen every day, but it may happen several times a week. Some mothers may find that it seems a common occurrence in the early evening hours or when a baby is teething. It is always helpful to remember that eventually your baby will outgrow this fussiness. In addition, some babies will be alert and awake for a long period of time although they will not be fussy in an uncomfortable sense. I believe that breastfed babies are more alert. Babies also need and want lots of cuddling and holding and the presence of their mothers. Fortunately, there are ways to soothe your baby without resorting to the pacifier. After all, women got along without them for years!

Here are some suggestions:

1. Carry your baby by using a cloth carrier or sling.

2. Make sure your baby is neither too cold nor too warm; many mothers tend to overdress a baby.

3. Offer the breast, or see first if your baby is interested by placing him in the nursing position. If he is not interested, you can offer the breast later. Your baby may refuse the breast initially and yet welcome it fifteen minutes later.

4. Rock, hold, carry, walk, sway, dance, or sing to your baby. Rub or pat his back. Try lying down on your back and placing your baby on top of you; the movements of your chest may comfort him. Your husband can be a help here when nursing isn't the answer.

5. Take a warm bath with your baby. Babies love to take baths with their mother. There's more physical contact and security for the baby, it's easier and more fun for the mother, and it has a relaxing effect upon both. You may find that afterwards your baby will nurse himself into a deep sleep.

6. Weather permitting, take baby for a walk outdoors. Baby slings and back carriers are ideal for this type of activity. Some parents leave home by car and hope a car ride helps an extremely fussy baby. For baby's safety, use a car seat in the back seat of the car. You can even learn to nurse the baby in the car seat when it is too inconvenient for your husband to stop the car.

7. Review the La Leche League manual, *The Womanly Art of Breastfeeding*, for helpful suggestions.[1]

There may be a time when nothing works. Friends who had colicky babies have told me that the best thing they did was to continue the 100% nursing and give them lots of the physical contact which all babies need. Their husband's help and support during this time was especially important to them. With most babies, the fussiness is brief, and normally a mother can find a more natural solution to baby's discomfort rather than using a pacifier. If you nap with your baby after lunch, you will also be in a better disposition to handle any fussiness that occurs later in the day.

"I have too much milk"

Most newborns will occasionally have difficulty handling the milk that comes from their mother's breast. The milk comes too fast, and the baby is inclined to fuss and pull away from the breast temporarily until the milk flow slows down. It is a situation more common for the baby in his early days or months. As he grows older, he will enjoy this ample supply. Other babies have satisfied their need for food but desire to nurse more. What they want is an empty breast, not one full of milk; so they react quite strongly when offered the other breast that is full.

There really isn't any problem in the first situation. The occasional time that this happens the mother can allow for more burping or wait until the letdown feeling — which is what causes the milk to come out so fast — has been completed. But don't wait if baby is crying. If baby is hungry, he'll be anxious to get back on the breast. So let him; if it's too much for him to handle again, he'll pull off and keep trying. If, however, this situation occurs at almost every feeding, you might find some of these ideas helpful.

1. Try a different nursing position, such as lying down. At night mothers seldom have this problem when sleeping with baby. Avoid using this "lying down" position for every feeding. One mother soon found that her baby would nurse only when lying down, and she found it was difficult to leave her home with this nursing baby.

2. Try offering your breast with your baby in a different nursing position so that the spray angles off to the side or top of your baby's mouth, if that's possible, to avoid having the spray go toward the back of his throat.

3. Offer only one breast at a feeding. This way your baby can satisfy his other sucking needs toward the end of the feeding on a breast that isn't full of milk. A small infant can receive plenty of milk from one breast at a feeding, especially when the supply is ample and the feedings are frequent. At the next feeding offer the other breast.

4. The mother who has a huge supply of milk might temporarily, during the early months, offer the same breast for approximately a two-hour period. In other words, you would feed your baby at 9:00 a.m. Then, if an hour later your baby wanted to nurse again, you would offer the same breast that you offered at 9:00. During the next two-hour period you would offer the other breast. This feeding pattern could be used until the milk supply settled and the baby could handle it better.

Normally, one-breast feedings with unrestricted and frequent nursing do not present any problem. However, since in using this method there is an increased risk of engorgement or a plugged duct with an abundant milk supply, the mother should be observant. If a breast becomes too full and drippy, you can express the excess milk by hand. If a tender spot is felt on the breast, you can let your baby suck on that breast as much as possible to keep it empty and usually the tenderness will disappear as quickly as it appeared. This is especially easy to do when sleeping with your baby during a nap or during the night. Any tender area of the breast should be quickly tended to.

Proper management of an overabundant milk supply may be a factor in the maintenance of infertility. For example, one mother wrote that she had so much milk that her four month old did not have to suckle; her milk just flowed into his mouth. She also felt this was why she had menstruated soon after childbirth. A few other mothers have also felt that an over-ample supply might have been the cause of an early return of menstruation following childbirth. The practices listed above to increase the amount of actual suckling, especially comfort nursing during the mother's sleep, may help these mothers postpone menstruation longer.

"We want to avoid thumbsucking"

Some parents offer the pacifier to avoid thumbsucking and possibly any future orthodontic expenses. Dentists hold varying opinions on the matter. In 1961 an orthodontist at the University of California School of Dentistry in San Francisco taught my class that 1) the young child should be allowed to suck his thumb if he desires and that parents should not discourage this habit until after the child is four years old; 2) thumbsucking will cause no harm to the permanent set of teeth if the child sucks up until four years of age; 3) the child's sucking needs are best satisfied at an early age when the child is allowed to nurse as much as he desires; and 4) breastfeeding satisfies this sucking need best. Regardless of various dentists' views about thumbsucking or pacifiers, most agree that suckling at the breast is better than sucking at bottles and pacifiers from the point of view of dental care.

Breastfeeding is a preventive measure against tongue thrusting. Tongue thrusting develops in an infant who pushes his tongue forward to slow down the fast flow of milk from a bottle and prevent the flooding of milk toward the back of the throat. I was a bottlefed baby and I was told in dental school that I had a slight tongue thrusting swallow, but not enough to cause any problems. Severe tongue thrusting, however, can interfere with speech and teeth alignment.

Mr. Daniel Garliner, a speech specialist who has lectured extensively to medical, dental and orthodontic groups in various parts of the United States and Canada, claims that we swallow 2,000 times a day! His point is that if a baby swallows incorrectly, he may later need speech therapy and dental correction. How do we prevent a deviate swallow or tongue thrusting in our children? Breastfeeding is the answer. Garliner says Mother Nature "designed the nursing act to be a forerunner of the speech act. Mothers were designed to nurse babies. It was imperative that the muscles of swallowing would receive sufficient exercises," so that "the infant would develop strong oral muscles." When the mother resorts to bottles and enlarged holes in the rubber nipple for speedy feedings, the fluid comes so quickly toward the back of his throat that the child has to protect himself. His only protection is his tongue which the baby uses to push forward. Once he learns this, a deviate swallow has developed.[2]

In the breastfeeding act, the baby has control of 1) "the length of the nipple, 2) the flow from the nipple, and 3) the flexibility of the nipple substance," according to Garliner in his book *Swallow Right— Or Else.* With artificial feeding, the baby loses control in these three areas. "There is no question that breastfeeding is the most desirable situation for the infant in terms of muscle development," says Garliner, and failure to provide a substitute for nature's system leads to "weakened facial musculature, more dental malocclusions, and speech defects."[3]

The stronger suckling required by breastfeeding involves a muscular action that promotes the proper growth and development of the jaw, bones, and muscular tissues of the entire face. Studies show that the presence of long-term nursing tends to decrease the need for orthodontic work. Breast-feeding is the first step in preventive orthodontics. Of course, orthodontic problems may arise from other factors that cannot be controlled by healthy suckling habits.

Both my husband and I were typical bottlefed babies, and we both required extensive orthodontic work as youngsters. None of our five breast-fed children, however, required any orthodontic work, a rare experience for a family in a neighborhood full of braces.

In studying the histories of 9,698 children, researchers at the Johns Hopkins School of Public Health found "that children bottlefed or breastfed for less than a year reported misaligned teeth 40% more often than children breastfed for more than one year... But those breastfed for three months or less and those who continued to suck a finger had the highest risk of crooked teeth." They concluded that breastfeeding contributes to straighter teeth because "it leads to different growth patterns in the mouth than those in bottlefed babies."[4]

Breastfeeding can reduce the risk of snoring and obstructive sleep apnea according to Brian Palmer, a dentist who has studied this topic for over 20 years. According to Palmer, the symptoms of obstructive sleep apnea are "loud snoring, daytime sleepiness, and interrupted sleep with periods of not breathing." Other symptoms for children include "headaches, hyperactivity, developmental delay, behavior problems, restless sleep, nightmares, bed wetting, and attention disorders." The best health practice for proper breathing during the night and for proper occlusion is "breastfeeding and keeping objects like pacifiers out of the mouth."[5]

The relationship between the use of the bottle as a pacifier and tooth decay has also been highlighted in the daily press and by dental organizations. What happens when the bottle is used as a pacifier? The contents of the bottle can seep into the mouth and bathe the teeth. An acquaintance of ours had this unpleasant experience happen to her eighteen month old, bottle-pacified child. This child needed his four front teeth capped due to dental decay and this capping required both hospitalization and the service of an anesthetist. The dentist explained that this decay was due to the lactic acid in the cow's milk used in the bottle.

Breastfeeding, especially lying-down nursing, is sometimes accused of causing this decay termed "nursing bottle syndrome." However, the act of obtaining milk when breastfeeding is completely different. The baby has to work for his milk and then swallows. If the baby falls asleep at the breast, there is no milk that pools around the teeth when he is not nursing. This important fact has been proven by a detailed study where combined pictures (motion pictures and radiography) showed that no milk accumulates in the mouth during nursing or after its cessation.[6] Dentist Louis M. Abbey, a professor of oral pathology at the Virginia Commonwealth University School of Dentistry, has studied the available literature on this subject and finds there is no convincing evidence which implicates the practice of unrestricted breastfeeding as a cause of early caries in infants.[7]

It must be remembered that dental decay is not caused by a single factor. The mother's diet and even her health during pregnancy can affect the formation of her child's teeth. The hygiene of her baby's teeth and his diet also influence the health of his teeth. For good dental hygiene, you can clean your child's teeth several times a day even when breastfeeding and avoid giving your baby sweets and highly refined foods. This is not meant to be a full discussion on oral hygiene but to show you that other factors come into play when discussing dental decay. In addition, our family dentist claims that the dental decay rate has been cut drastically since Cincinnati added fluoride to the drinking water. He is seeing many more youngsters today who are cavity-free.

On the other hand, we know that some breastfed babies do develop decay on their front teeth. I nursed four of our children with lying-down and extended nursing. Three had no sign of front tooth decay but one did. With this fourth child, Karen, I had a fever during the pregnancy that probably affected the developing tooth buds. We were thankful for a dentist who, from his experience with his own children, preferred the conservative approach. Prior to kindergarten one of Karen's lateral teeth began to bother her, and our family dentist recommended a pediatric oral surgeon. Since the other lateral tooth was very similar in appearance, she had both removed. The experience was such a pleasant one that she wanted to go back to have her ugly central incisors removed as well. One of the reasons for this was that the parent was allowed to stay until the child was asleep in the chair.

I continued the breastfeeding during those early years when her upper four teeth were eroding because our dentist never told me to wean. I nursed Karen and two other children for four to five years; the other two children had excellent dental health. I also appreciated the fact that our family dentist did not insist on hospitalization and treatment at an early age. The decay was such that we were able to wait and treat the situation at a much later date as necessary. Our dentist saw her on a regular basis. I might add that this child is now an adult with beautiful healthy teeth.

My advice to mothers who find themselves in similar situations is to continue nursing but consult several dentists, if that's what it takes, until you find one who is good with children and tends to take a conservative approach. When we moved to Cincinnati, I visited three dentists for regular dental care before I found one who I felt would be good with children. In addition, although our child's upper front teeth looked bad, treatment could wait for three to four years, and the central incisors fell out naturally. However, there will be other cases where the decayed teeth should be treated immediately. Parents should not neglect the care of their children's teeth.

Dentist Harry Torney studied all the research on breastfeeding and dental decay.[8] He found the most significant factors contributing to dental decay in breastfed babies were: 1) defective enamal, 2) mother's illness during pregnancy, 3) mother's stressful pregnancy, such as bereavement, and 4) mothers tended to take three times less dairy products during pregnancy.

Pacifier problems

Pacifiers may be dangerous objects. Some may break into pieces which can cut or choke a baby. They can also be a ready source of germs. An acquaintance from Brazil told me that the mothers all nursed their children but that they also used bottles and pacifiers. He spoke of their poor sanitation, and he was especially concerned about the various types of worms the child could ingest by sucking on a dirty pacifier. Government regulations can reduce design and manufacturing problems but obviously can do nothing about hygiene.

Heavy use of pacifiers may delay speech or cause speech problems. I remember trying to converse with a toddler who was not responsive due to the pacifier in his mouth. His mother said that he didn't talk because the pacifier was usually in his mouth. Some children talk with pacifiers in their mouth, but they are very hard to understand. A speech clinic on a college campus analyzed its speech cases and discovered that 80% to 90% of their childhood speech cases were due to excessive and extended use of the pacifier or bottle. The pacifier was used by the parent to quiet the child, and as a result the child suffered from a lack of conversation and had speech difficulties. The problem occurred more frequently in homes where both parents were working. Forty-four percent of the children with speech problems came from homes where both parents worked while only twenty-five percent came from homes where a single parent lived. The two working parents talked to each other after work and let their child watch television, but the single parent talked to his/her child after work for companionship.[9]

Pacifiers may create breastfeeding problems for the nursing mother. They were well described in a La Leche League publication by a counseling mother.

> It happened again, and I am finally moved to write. A mother called with a six-month-old baby on a nursing strike. Among other things I asked if she used a pacifier with her baby. I was almost sure the answer would be "yes," and it was. This is getting to be one of my routine counseling questions. When a mother with a one-month-old calls because her baby

isn't gaining weight, or a mother calls because her three-month-old seems to be going through a growth spurt but will only nurse while the milk freely flows, nine times out of ten these babies suck long and frequently on pacifiers.

Perhaps I am so aware of this because heavy pacifier use was one of the downfalls in nursing our firstborn. He, too, nursed only for milk and got his main comfort from the pacifier. He would never nurse at length to build up a greater supply; during growth spurts I added extra solid food. By five months the nursing just petered out.

Even if the situation never gets this drastic, isn't one of the joys of nursing found in being your own baby's "pacifier"? To be able to soothe your little one at the breast when he needs this comforting form of love is one of the nicest inherent advantages of breastfeeding.[10]

Shortened lactation

Pacifiers can definitely shorten lactation. A study in Brazil looked at 600 babies to determine if pacifier use at the age of one month affected breast-feeding at the age of six months. At one month of age, 55% of the babies were using pacifiers, and 23% were using them "during the whole day and at night to help them fall asleep (or even while sleeping)." The remaining 32% were classified as partial users. The researchers concluded that those infants using pacifiers at one month of age were "three times more likely to be weaned at six months of age." They warned against using pacifiers since they are associated with early weaning.[11] Since mothers in this study were using pacifiers to get the baby to sleep, I have to add here that the easiest way to get your baby to sleep is to nurse him to sleep.

Breastfeeding is often a form of comfort nursing. The baby can some-times fill up in a few minutes at the breast, but there are many times, especially when tired, that he will need to be pacified at the breast. You can see how soothing the breast is for comfort when you allow your baby to remain there. The breast may even bring comfort to a bottlefed baby. One mother told me about her adopted baby who was extremely fussy and nothing worked in her efforts to quiet him down. She had not intended to nurse this baby even though she had nursed her other children. But out of desperation, she offered the breast. To her surprise, it worked. She continued to bottlefeed but used the breast to soothe her baby and as an aid to sleep.

Early return of fertility

The absence of pacifiers may be crucial in the maintenance of natural infertility. Nature provided the baby with his mother's breast and with his own fingers for satisfying his sucking needs. Artificial devices replace nature's products — and, as we have seen, the absence of natural mothering usually means the reduction of nursing at the breast and therefore the absence or shortening of natural child spacing. The two — natural mothering and natu-ral child spacing — go together.

The following two stories illustrate that exclusive breastfeeding does not assure breastfeeding infertility since both mothers nursed exclusively for a considerable length of time and yet both experienced menstrual periods while doing so. However, their babies did use the pacifier regularly.

One mother had two periods by the time she was five months postpartum and while exclusively nursing. She told me this while her second child was cradled in her arms, sucking on a pacifier. We began to talk about pacifiers and how babies learn to suck on them instead of the breast. I then related this to the importance of the suckling act for the natural suppression of fertility. She said she had nursed her first baby although not exclusively. Yet with him, up to the age of her present five month old, she had not menstruated; she had never given her first baby a pacifier.

Another friend nursed her baby for seven months before introducing solids but experienced regular periods after childbirth. She nursed her baby every three and a half to four hours and offered him a pacifier so she "wouldn't have to nurse the baby all the time." Interestingly, this mother had several periods and then missed two periods during the time she was expressing milk for another baby in addition to feeding her own baby. Maybe this extra stimulation suppressed her fertility, for her periods resumed after she no longer expressed the extra milk for the other baby and was once again providing only for her own. The addition of the comfort nursing might also have suppressed her menstruation.

Does the pacifier make the difference? It certainly can, as these anecdotes illustrate. If the babies in the above stories had been pacified as well as fed at the breast, maybe the additional suckling might have provided breastfeeding's natural infertility.

Thumbsucking

The absence of pacifiers automatically leads to the subject of thumbsucking, a subject which deserves more consideration and study with respect to mothering. Dr. James Clark Moloney, writing in *Child and Family* magazine,[12] discussed pathological thumbsucking and attempted to show that the baby who sucks his thumb may be "mothering" himself; the thumb may become a substitute for the mother's breast and body. He explained how mother-body contact and free access to the breast provide satisfaction and reassurance to the infant, and how such an infant has no need for a substitute. Noting other cultures, he told of the Okinawan mother who places her baby at the breast immediately after birth and continues to remain in close touch with him. The child is carried on his mother's back, and she caresses and cuddles him. The child sleeps on a mat with his parents. He is allowed to creep and crawl and explore on his own, yet he knows he can return to his mother's side any time he desires. The baby is so closely related to his mother that she senses his needs before he cries. He pointed out that unfortunately many American mothers tend to minister to their infants and then set them aside and leave them, treating them in what he

27

called an undesirable arm's-length manner. Our culture tends to produce thumbsuckers since maternal intimacy is lacking.

It is obvious that excessive thumbsucking can have the same effect as a pacifier on the natural spacing processes in some cases, so some mothers have felt very strongly that the baby should not suck his thumb or fingers at all. I cannot be as strong about this issue. A few babies will suck their fingers often in spite of frequent nursing and close contact with mother. Babies may want to suck temporarily when uncomfortable — during a burping session or in a car ride when mother is driving and can't respond — and they will begin to suck upon awakening from their sleep as hunger develops. This sucking signals a need to his mother who can offer the breast before he is fully awake and before he cries. Rather obviously, she will have to be physically close to him to notice such needs.

Physical closeness makes the mother more aware of her child's needs — so much so that it is the key requirement for natural spacing. Natural mothering, with its physical mother-baby closeness and unrestricted nursing, does not come easily in our society. With little outside support, most of us have learned the "art of mothering" by caring for several babies. I admire and almost envy the young mother who has all this information before the birth of her first child. She can adopt this type of mothering right away and receive the joys that come from it in her first effort. Some of us have felt that we did a good job of mothering only to discover that with our next child we were doing things a bit differently. We mature and learn with each child. The difference may be slight, but it appears to be enough to eliminate the thumbsucking in some cases. Table I shows how three children were raised, each a little differently, by one mother.

May I quote the mother's remarks about thumbsucking with her children?

> [Our first child] started sucking his fingers fairly early but I don't remember exactly when. He spontaneously gave this up when he was about 4½ years old or a little more. [Our second child] started sucking her thumb before she was a year old and became quite an inveterate thumbsucker. At 4½ she still sucks it a lot, chiefly at night or when tired or upset. I think our children must have a tremendous sucking need, and although I was more free in nursing this second child, and she in fact nursed a lot more than "average," it was obviously not enough to prevent the thumbsucking. [Our third child] is by far the most independent of our three, and the only one who has never sucked her thumb or fingers. I have the feeling that if it weren't for so much nursing she would definitely have been a thumbsucker. Occasionally I have seen her put her thumb in her mouth and start to half-suck, and then I would always pick her up for a nursing.

It is interesting to note that as this mother gradually developed a more natural mothering style with each child, her length of postpartum infertility also increased.

I do not want to give the impression that anything more than the tiniest bit of thumbsucking will destroy the ecological balance. It happens on occasion that a mother who adopts the natural mothering style may still have a baby who sucks his fingers or thumbs without the mother having an early return of fertility. It is likewise true that some thumbsuckers with extremely frequent, unrestricted and prolonged nursing will stop sucking their fingers at a later date and then use only the breast for pacification.

Table I:
Different Styles of Mothering and Their Effects on Fertility

	CHILD #1	CHILD #2	CHILD #3
PACIFIER	For only 3 months	None	None
BOTTLE	Gave 72 ounces during early post-partum weeks; mother had serious breast infections	None	None
SOLIDS BEGUN	At 6 months; with spoon	At 6 months; with spoon	At 9 months; with finger foods
CUP BEGUN	At 9 months; mother offered cup	After one year; on his own	After one year; on his own
NURSING COMPLETED	At 16 months	At 27 months	Still nursing at 28 months
NIGHT FEEDINGS	First 6 months; then baby slept through	First 6 months; then baby slept through	Still nurses at night at 28 months
SLEEPING ARRANGEMENT	In the crib	Mother nursed baby in bed but returned to crib	In parents' bed
PERIODS RESUMED	At 12 months postpartum	At 18 months postpartum	Never did; reduced nursings to achieve pregnancy, which occurred 27 months postpartum
THUMB-SUCKING	3 months to 4-1/2 years	From 1 year to more than 4-1/2 years	Absent

The point I am emphasizing is that mothering practices in which the mother personally takes care of the nutritional and emotional sucking needs of the infant are those which reinforce the mother-baby ecology and tend to postpone the return of fertility and menstruation. The mother who adopts the philosophy of physical closeness and who has her baby physically near her at night as well as during the day is in a position to recognize the various sucking needs of her infant. When she satisfies these needs at the breast, she cooperates with the natural pattern. Offering the breast when she notices her baby sucking his thumb or fingers not only provides some milk and emotional comfort, it also may reduce or prevent a habit of thumbsucking from birth or at a later date. Some of my correspondents have been quite emphatic on this whole subject, and some have stated their plans to offer the breast more with a future child when they see him sucking his thumb. You have the choice and can benefit from the accumulated experience. Remember that with the frequent and unrestricted nursing of the natural mothering program, thumbsucking is usually absent.

Other soothers

The childcare industry has come up with any number of things that can be used as mother substitutes. Used to excess, these items not only interfere with the mother-baby ecology of breastfeeding and natural infertility, but they can also hinder the child's development. For example, hospitals have found that infants need tender, loving care and that infants deprived of this care and physical contact will wither and not develop normally. The classic story is about an orphanage where infants, kept in cribs, were given adequate nutrition and sanitation but where there was a high rate of unexplained sickness and subnormal progress and development — except the babies near the door. Finally it was realized that the babies near the door were getting little bits of extra attention from nurses and maids as they came in and out of the door — patting them on the head, speaking to them, and so forth. From such examples we can see that a crib or a playpen could be used in such a way that it becomes a prison instead of a temporary protection against falling or getting hurt in some way.

Some mothers in the past practically worshipped the infant seat. They wouldn't let anyone pick up the baby, so a piece of equipment became his habitual home. Now this has been replaced by the movable car seat. One device that is most easy to use to excess is the swing seat. Just place the baby in the seat, and baby may be content, almost hypnotically, for literally hours. One former neighbor bragged about the fact that her baby ate and slept in such a swing.

Strollers can also be used in a similar manner when the mother is busy at a conference or shopping. My friend and I observed a baby at a conference who remained in the stroller the entire day; he even fed himself from a bottle while remaining in the stroller. I don't think it requires much imagination to see how such baby care practices result in greatly reduced mother-baby contacts and reduced breastfeeding, thus upsetting the ecology of breastfeeding and natural infertility. Equipment should never replace mother. Babies thrive when you hold them and keep them physically close to you.

Attitudes can change. With our first baby we thought a playpen was an absolute necessity, but we rarely used it. Our baby did not like it. We lost it in a move and never replaced it. Many devices can be temporarily helpful to the mother. For example, a playpen under the shade of a tree might be used for a short time while the parents are working in the garden. Some equipment might be temporarily enjoyable for the baby to use. Unfortunately parents often use these items more and more as a substitute for the parenting they should be doing.

Another mother who questions the use of pacifiers and other equipment as mother-substitutes is Dr. Karen Walant. This psychotherapist speaks unkindly about many of our parenting practices which she considers to be abusive because they promote "separation, self-soothing and detachment at the expense of attachment, intimacy, and connectedness." She criticizes the use of pacifiers so a baby does not need his mother. She believes that babies should be addicted to their mothers and not to their pacifiers. "Babies need to be held — as much as possible, as often as possible. Therefore, I consider the over-use of strollers, playpens, and even cribs to be normative abuse." By normative, she is referring to practices which "appear normal for our culture."[13]

I believe that the absence of the pacifier and over-used baby items can make a big difference in the job of parenting as well. Joy comes in the giving when we don't rely on these items. Parenting is more enjoyable and more rewarding for both mom and dad when they learn to comfort their baby by themselves. You have closer contact with your child as you calm him down without resorting to other gadgets. There is nothing more satisfying than to have spent some time settling your baby and then to have your baby fall asleep on your shoulder or chest or in your arms. Maybe 15 minutes ago you were anxious to pass the job on to someone else due to fatigue. Then after your child falls asleep in your arms, you're reluctant to put him down! You find yourself wanting to hold your child a little longer and to take a few extra minutes to enjoy this little precious person.

One piece of equipment that keeps mother and baby together, and can be used by dad, is the baby carrier. I have used front cloth carriers and back carriers with all five children. They are most helpful and invaluable for this natural form of mothering. For newborns and small babies less than six months old, a cloth carrier is recommended so that the baby can be carried on mother's front. In some societies mothers use cloth carriers to carry their babies on their back. A cloth carrier can be made very inexpensively, and it provides the same support as considerably more expensive manufactured cloth carriers.[14] In contrast with other devices, baby carriers are not mother substitutes but actually help to provide the same closeness given by similar carriers among the more nature-oriented peoples of the world.

The Second Standard of pacifying your baby at the breast is crucial if you want to enjoy the side benefit of natural infertility. As we have seen, this type of mothering at the breast has many benefits for the baby, and I believe it is much more rewarding for parents.

The third standard

Don't use bottles and pacifiers. This standard means that you do not offer your baby any food or liquid in a bottle (or a cup) during the first six months of life nor do you give your baby a pacifier. This standard is implicit in the first two standards dealing with exclusive breastfeeding and pacification of the baby at the breast.

One of the most common remarks made to nursing mothers among those in the medical profession is this negative question: "You don't want to be a pacifier to your baby, do you?" This implies that the baby is always at the breast, especially today when it is so common to see a baby with a pacifier almost always in his mouth. The inference is clearly that if the pacifier is always in the baby's mouth, then certainly he will want the breast to be always in his mouth. Of course, this is not the case.

It also implies that you do not want to comfort your baby. Pacification at the breast is a form of comfort nursing, and certainly as a mother you would want to comfort your baby through breastfeeding as nature intended.

Most mothers do not offer a cup to their baby prior to six months. An emergency situation is something else. But under normal circumstances, cup feeding is not necessary during the first six months of life.

Bottles are not necessary either in normal situations. Because the use of bottles is so common today, I re-emphasize that they are unnecessary when you are present to your baby and are breastfeeding. This also applies to bottles of your own milk.

The third standard is included to add the emphasis needed in our bottlefeeding culture and to help you visualize that these items are not needed. In most cases you can do a good job of parenting a baby without them when you follow the ecological breastfeeding program.

[1] See Mini-Catalog at back of book.
[2] Daniel Garliner, *Your Swallow: An Aid to Dental Health*, self-published.
[3] D. Garliner, *Swallow Right — Or Else*, St. Louis: Warren H. Green, 1979.
[4] *The New York Times*, "Breastfeeding Linked to Straighter Teeth," June 2, 1987.
[5] Brian Palmer, "Breastfeeding: Reducing the Risk for Obstructive Sleep Apnea," *Breastfeeding Abstracts*, February 1999.
[6] G.M. Ardan et al., "A Cineradiographic Study of Breastfeeding," *Br. J. Radiol.*, March 1958, 156.
[7] L.M. Abbey, "Is Breastfeeding a Likely Cause of Dental Caries in Young Children?" JADA, 98, January 1979, 21.

[8] Harry Torney, "Breastfeeding and Dental Health," 1995 La Leche League International Conference.

[9] Carol Innerst, "Popping Pacifier in Tot's Mouth May Retard Speech Development," *The Washington Times*, November 15, 1991.

[10] *Leaven*, May-June 1972.

[11] F. Barros, C. Victoria, T. Semer, S. Filho, E. Tomasi, and E. Weiderpass, "Use of Pacifiers is Associated with Decreased Breastfeeding," *Pediatrics*, April 1995, 497-99.

[12] J.C. Moloney, "Thumbsucking," *Child and Family*, Summer 1967.

[13] Karen Walnut, "Fostering Healthy Attachment," *The Nurturing Parent,* Summer 1996.

[14] A homemade front sling for your baby is easy to make and no sewing is required. Take 2½ yards of sturdy fabric, 36 inches wide, and tie the ends together in a double knot. Wear it as a sling over one shoulder and across your chest with the knot in back; you can put it on or remove it without untying the knot. Your baby will fit securely in front because the material tucks in around his buttocks and offers support for his head. Extra material gathered around his shoulders can be pulled up over his head to provide protection on an extremely windy or sunny day. A pattern for a cloth sling can frequently be purchased at a fabric store. Back baby carriers for older babies can be purchased at department stores, baby stores, and camping stores.

5

New Light on Night Feedings

THE FOURTH STANDARD:
Sleep with your baby for night feedings.

This topic does not appeal to many parents, but it's an important one to consider if you are interested in the natural child spacing effect of breast-feeding. Night feedings are normal for a breastfed baby. Many infants need one or several feedings nightly during the first few years of life. These feedings are important for several reasons, the most obvious being that they form a part of the baby's nutrition. In fact, some doctors will be concerned for nutritional reasons if your small baby is sleeping through the night. Second, the regularity of nursing during the night produces a regular supply of milk. Third, night feedings are important because the frequent and unre-stricted nursing which maintains an ample milk supply is also responsible for the natural spacing. A mother who anticipates that her breastfeeding will result in both a healthy baby and natural infertility will not go for 10 to 12 hours without nursing during the day. She should likewise not set a goal of so many hours without nursing her baby during the night. The absence of a feeding for any length of time may initiate an early return of your menstrual periods and thereby shorten your breastfeeding infertility. If you want the natural child spacing effect of breastfeeding, then sleep with your baby and give your baby the night feedings he will naturally desire.

Contemporary social attitudes

Contemporary emphasis is placed on getting the baby to sleep all the way through the night and at the earliest possible date. The longer the baby sleeps at night, the better he is thought to be. Parents pride themselves on how soon they can get their new baby to sleep the entire night. They fill up the baby before bedtime with the hope that this will satisfy him for the duration of the night. If the baby does wake, they hope that the fussing or crying will only be temporary, so that they will not have to get out of bed — for which no one can blame them. When those hopes fail and they have to get up, they might have to go to the bother of warming up a bottle; and by the time that chore is done — to the tune of the baby's crying — all they are hoping for is that the baby will feed himself back to sleep without further

35

ado. Maybe the baby needs burping and that means a second trip from bed to baby. With this type of routine, it's no wonder that bottlefeeding parents aim for that goal of "all through the night as early as possible."

Others hope to do the trick with the pacifier. As one mother put it rather bluntly, "Let's face it. We stick the pacifier back in their mouths, hoping they'll settle down and go back to sleep again." Another answer to the problem was given by a doctor to a friend of mine. He told the couple to put the baby in the bathroom, close the door, and let the baby cry it out.

The breastfeeding mother is often instructed to wean the baby from night feedings at an early age. If her baby objects, she is often advised to ignore his cries. She may be told to offer him a bottle or to let her husband take care of the baby because all the baby wants is his mother anyway! One mother we know was advised by her doctor to give her two-month-old baby a drug so he would sleep through the night. At any rate, most babies sleep away from their mothers in our society, and they eventually learn to sleep through the night on their own. These babies never have the pleasure of receiving from their mother and father during the night hours that touch stimulation said to be so important.

Our society can be very cruel to parents who share sleep with their baby. One young mother who took our natural family planning classes came up to thank my husband and me for teaching them because the natural mothering had made such an impact on their lives as parents. She and her husband had recently returned from visiting her relatives over Thanksgiving. The dinner was ruined when the relatives found out they were sleeping with their five-month-old baby while visiting, and they received criticism throughout the meal.

Unfortunately our society seems to condone parental non-involvement. "Give them a drink. Put them to bed and leave." Most recently, more and more parents are relying on television to get their little ones to sleep. Dr. Robert Lerer, a county health commissioner in the Greater Cincinnati area, was saddened to learn that one-third of one year olds and two-thirds of two year olds fall asleep watching TV or a video. And one-fourth of these children fall asleep in front of the television set every night![1]

Obviously parents should be more involved with their small children at bedtime. Besides the breastfeeding, nighttime activities can include rocking, reading, walking, praying, singing, storytelling, and even bed-sharing. These activities are more likely to occur with the natural mothering and parenting program. Nursing a small child to sleep early in the evening requires little effort or extra time. Many nights I talked with my husband as I rocked and nursed a little one to sleep in the rocking chair. Depending on their age I would either place them nearby or else would take them to bed when they fell asleep. When we lived in Salina, Kansas a friend often dropped by in the evening to visit us. She was simply amazed to see how easily Margaret fell asleep at the breast while she, my husband and I were enjoying each other's company. Margaret at that time was two years old. This friend was so impressed with the ease of nursing a little one to sleep that she had to tell others, including the dentists for whom she worked. I did not have to walk the floor with her, nor spend time getting her water or coaxing her to go to bed. Breastfeeding was such an easy lifestyle for nighttime sleeping.

Personal Experience

The problem of night feeding is partially eliminated by a change of attitudes, by simply looking to the best interests of the baby instead of to our own convenience. During my first three years of mothering, I had frequent contact with a small group of women who placed a great deal of emphasis on the needs of their babies. I read many of their recommended books. These mothers belonged to La Leche League, a group that offers correct breastfeeding information plus support. In the United States, most successful nursing mothers since the Sixties have had some contact with the League. Their influence has been profound, even in the formation of The Couple to Couple League.

During my early mothering years, I learned that good mothering meant meeting baby's needs during the night as well as during the day. Therefore, it was common to hear a mother speak of night feedings when her child was 12 months old or even 18 months old. When we moved, I soon learned that such a group was in the minority, that most people have entirely different views about raising children compared to those views I had acquired from my original exposure. In our new environment, it seemed that the question most frequently asked about our baby was: "Is she sleeping through the night now?" or "How often do you have to feed her during the night?" According to this viewpoint, night feedings are a problem to be eliminated instead of an ordinary part of childcare.

The answer to such questions is rather simple. Our children will never take a prize for all-night sleeping at an early age. My husband and I learned eventually that this is one phase they will outgrow when they are ready. Not only are there many advantages to both parent and baby in letting nature take its course in this area, but doing so eliminates all the worries and problems inherent in training a child to sleep through the night.

Our first two children awoke for night feedings every night until we decided that it might be time to stop this "habit." When they were both 18 months old, we tried all the tricks and none worked. So we resorted to the "crying it out" scheme. That worked within two or three nights. We would never do it this way again if we had another chance, but at that time we were uninformed and slow learners. We didn't feel this was the best way, but we conformed to our society's norms and thus made our children also conform.

With our second child I discovered, and then my husband learned, that sleeping with the baby was safe, and we were becoming more open to the philosophy of the family bed. We grew even more with our third child. The family bed was a reality from the day of her birth, and we adopted the

37

natural mothering/parenting lifestyle by following a more natural, child-centered approach. Accepting the family bed with our second baby was the first step that led us to accept changes in other areas of parenting. This book would have never been written if we had remained a two-child family.

While our intentions were right, sometimes it is more difficult to adjust to the family bed as the child turns one or two years old. My husband was slow to accept the family bed when our third child, then two years old, was still in our bed. He insisted one night that she stay in a separate bed and placed her alone in a separate room. He closed the door to soften the cries. The crying began, but it didn't last long. Our oldest daughter (then six years old) brought her to our bed since she couldn't stand it any longer, and the youngest stayed for many more nights. At four years of age she was sleeping through the night in her own bed in a room shared with two siblings. We were living in a two bedroom apartment at that time.

Sometimes parents can be in doubt about this practice. Well past her third birthday, our third child was still crawling into bed with us at some time during the wee hours for some nursing. When we had our doubts, support came in one form or another.

Some of this support came in the form of writings which I will refer to later. Other support came through personal acquaintances and correspondence. I learned from a friend that her child, although weaned when 10 months old, didn't sleep naturally through the night until she was 4½ years old. From other mothers, I learned that many have a similar situation at night, regardless of whether they chose to bottlefeed or breastfeed. However, since babies are "supposed" to sleep through the night, many mothers do not admit it nor do they like to talk about it. Likewise, I was fortunate to be able to correspond with other nursing mothers, and I found that there was always someone else who was night-nursing a baby older than ours. You can't imagine how much support this was!

Our last three children were in bed with us during the entire night for two years. Then we had a very slow transition period that lasted another two to three years. The transition over these years was so slow and gradual that it was very uneventful and happened almost without notice. They are all good sleepers and none of our five children have had sleeping or bedwetting problems. We are pleased with the results. In our experience, taking care of the child's real needs at this early stage does not set a pattern for the development of an emotionally unstable child. Quite the opposite occurs. They **do** outgrow that need to be with mom and dad during the night. Our child who was still coming in during the night at age 3½ was, a year later, not only sleeping all through the night but was the last one to wake up in the morning!

Bedtime was not rigid in our household. If a child took a late nap and was wide-awake at his usual bedtime, we would allow her or him to remain up. But they were not allowed to be active. They could only do quiet activities which usually limited them to reading or looking at books. If we were having fun with other families late in the evening, we did not say "Oh, it's 8:00. Time for them to be in bed!" and then leave. We stayed and enjoyed the activities. I feel sorry for children whose parents revolve the day's schedule around their children's sleep. The child's sleeping becomes the top priority of the day so the parent or parents can get other things done. Babies and children will get sleepy, but life or living should not be set around a goal of sleeping at such and such a time and for so long. Attitudes about sleep are usually healthier with natural parenting.

How to feed your baby at night

Nighttime feedings are no bother when mothers nurse in bed and fall asleep while doing so. "Horrors! What kind of a mother would admit to falling asleep while nursing her baby in bed? What if she rolls over on her baby?" These are common fears expressed by doctors, nurses, and acquaintances. These are fears that I also had with our first child. I heard about the advantages of nursing in bed, but I still couldn't overcome my fears to give it a try. I'd sit in a chair for the night feedings and was often cold and tired. After fifteen or twenty minutes of nursing, I would take the baby off the breast even though she wanted to suckle more in her sleep. I wanted to nurse her as quickly as possible so I could get back to bed myself.

With our next baby, a nursing mother again encouraged me to try nursing the baby in bed. I was a very tired mother, but this was advice I could 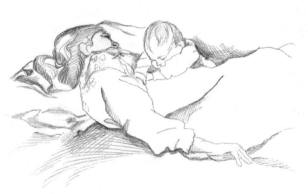 not accept. However, one afternoon I was so tired I fell asleep when nursing the baby in bed. Three hours later I awoke to find the baby still at the breast. And to my surprise, she was safe and still sleeping. I was well rested and felt wonderful. What a convenience!

I find that other nursing mothers are also reluctant to give it a try. They have these same acquired fears. Eventually some of them do give it a try, and then they begin to rave about the advantages of lying down to nurse the baby.

The fact that there is a natural instinct to protect your baby cannot be ignored. This is a good thing. Certainly, you must make sure comforters or pillows are not near his face and avoid the soft wavy waterbeds. Obviously anything soft, such as bean bags, are not to be used. The baby may be dressed in a warm trundle bundle so that he can lie on top of the blankets. Our babies were always tucked under the blankets with the sheets and blankets below their face. After nursing, their heads turned away from the breast or toward the top of the bed. We kept our babies usually in the center of the bed between us so they would not fall off. I learned to offer both breasts during the night without changing the baby's position. If I nursed an older child in a double bed with a sibling, I would put a piece of furniture next to the side of the bed to prevent the little one from falling out of bed. Beds can also be placed up against the wall or various sleeping arrangements can be made on the floor. One young mother had a good idea. She and her husband had wall-to-wall beds in one bedroom; the other bedroom was used for chest of drawers and for toys. Sleeping arrangements do not have to be expensive. Sometimes a sturdy foam cot or sleeping bag or combination will do.

If the father is a light sleeper, the baby can sleep on the other side of his mother, near the side of the bed. When the baby is small, a chair or his own bed can be placed at the side of the parents' bed to prevent him from falling. Having a big, roomy bed, such as a king-size, is an asset to this type of program. When purchasing a larger bed, consider the future savings from breastfeeding and from your not having to buy a baby crib, and remember: you do not need a headboard or a footboard.

Some mothers find it difficult to nurse lying down at first. One mother preferred a comfortable lounge chair for night feedings. Whichever way you choose, the important thing during the night is to be physically close enough to your child to sense his needs and to allow your child to nurse without interruption or at his leisure without your getting tired. You will learn how to take care of your baby's needs during the night while you sleep, and you will be well rested in the morning. Needless to say, if a mother has been drinking heavily or has been taking sleeping pills or is incapacitated in some way with a mind-altering substance, she should not take the baby to bed with her that night.

The advantages of bed-sharing

In normal situations, bed-sharing with your little one is much safer statistically than having your baby sleeping in a crib. The risk of SIDS (Sudden Infant Death Syndrome) is very low in countries where bed-sharing among parents and little ones is common. Lois Rogers, a medical writer, listed some interesting statistics worldwide concerning SIDS and stressed that these deaths could be avoided or reduced by simply having the mothers sleep with their babies. "Leading scientists have found that unexplained infant death — when babies simply stop breathing and die in their sleep — is virtually unknown across 95% of the world, where infants generally sleep close to their mothers." She states that SIDS is practically unheard of in India; among Asian babies 24 out of 25 sleep with their mother. Despite poverty and overcrowding, these Asian babies have a much lower cot death rate than Britain where one-third of the babies sleep alone. In spite of the campaign for babies to sleep on their back in Britain, there are still between 400 to 500 cot deaths a year there. Britain's infant cot death rate or SIDS rate is 23 times higher than Hong Kong where bed-sharing is common.[2] Another writer, Bill Manson, stressed the reduction of SIDS and the fact that babies would be happier and healthier if parents slept with their babies. Where it is customary for babies to share sleep with their parents (Hong Kong, Pakistan, Japan, and Bangladesh), the SIDS rates are very low compared to the United States, Britain, Canada, Australia and New Zealand where co-sleeping is uncommon. Manson showed how babies do not get smothered; healthy babies will scream the minute they get pinched or crowded.[3] Having had an original fear of smothering my baby in bed, I can truthfully say that during the 14-plus years that we practiced the family bed, I never experienced this "smothering" fear after we began co-sharing sleep with our babies. Nothing protects a baby 100% from cot death, including the family bed. But statistically a baby is safer in the family bed than in a crib.

Parents are encouraged today to have their babies sleep on their backs. When I first heard this, I thought of the benefit of nursing the baby in the family bed. With bed-sharing the infant usually ends up sleeping on his back or side because that is the position he is in when nursing and when he is finished nursing. Bed-sharing with breastfeeding almost automatically provides the position recommended as a protective measure against SIDS.

Another protective factor against SIDS is that co-sharing sleep improves the breathing development of the baby. This was brought to parents' attention back in the mid-1900s. Dr. Margaret Ribble, in her 1943 book, *The Rights of Infant,*[4] explained the various factors that can hamper a baby's breathing after birth and asked how a mother can facilitate her baby's breathing. The answer: sleep with her baby. As she said, the mother furnishes the "stimulus which is necessary to bring important reflex mechanisms into action. It so happens that the baby's first response to her touch is respiratory... From being held, fondled, allowed to suck freely and frequently, the child receives reflex stimulation, which primes his breathing mechanisms into action and which finally enables the whole respiratory process to become organized under the control of his own nervous system." She noted that many women still fear that they will suffocate their baby, but she said the exact opposite is true. In her own words, the mother's contact as her child sleeps at her side "is a protection rather than a peril." After explaining the importance of the establishment of the respiratory system on the development of other areas of the body, she concluded: "The importance of mothering in helping the child to breathe at this time can hardly be stressed too greatly," and "the quiet baby has to be watched with special care." In essence, mother's presence or breathing can act as a "pacemaker" for the baby's breathing.

What Dr. Ribble taught has been confirmed by current research, especially that conducted by Dr. James McKenna. This doctor claims that sleeping with the baby may prevent some of the cases of SIDS that strike one out of 500 American babies and is the leading killer of this nation's babies ages one month to one year.[5] When napping with his son, Dr. McKenna noticed that his baby's breathing pattern changed with his own. This experience led anthropologist McKenna to monitor the breathing patterns and other vital signs of a parent and baby as they slept in separate rooms, as they slept in the same room, and as they slept in the same bed. Evidence indicated that the baby's breathing pattern followed the mother's when they slept together but not when they slept apart. With SIDS, babies stop breathing for no apparent reason and, according to him, 90% of these cases occur in babies younger than six months. McKenna explains that human breathing patterns change between the second and the fourth months of life in preparation for speech, and he speculates that SIDS would be reduced by bedsharing and the infants picking up cues from their parents that would help their breathing systems to mature. Interestingly, this doctor was involved in a study which concluded "that infants who bedshare routinely at home breastfeed three times longer during the night than the infants who routinely sleep separately."[6] The greatly increased amount of nursing when the baby sleeps with his mother during the night obviously influences the effectiveness of the natural spacing mechanism.

I've already said that the nursing mother finds that she can satisfy her child's needs with little inconvenience or loss of sleep. Being so close to her child, the mother can wake up temporarily at his first stir to offer the breast. The child does not have to stir and stir and then finally cry to get her attention as he would if he were in a separate room. Even the dad can tap mom on the shoulder if he notices the baby mouthing or rooting for food during the night. After offering the breast, the mother then dozes back to sleep. This becomes so easy and natural that a mother cannot say how many times she nursed during the night. Nursing your baby is one job you can do well in your sleep.

The American Academy of Pediatrics is now encouraging parents to respond to their babies before the crying begins. In their Breastfeeding Policy Statement only two words were printed in boldface and italics. One was "late", as used in the following sentence. "Crying is a *late* indicator of hunger."[7] Rooting, mouthing, and increased activity or alertness are the earlier signs of hunger to which parents should respond. With the family bed you and your husband can respond to these earlier signs of hunger during the night because of the physical closeness to your baby.

Another advantage of bedsharing is the restfulness a mother can derive from nursing in bed or lying down for a nap. In fact, mothers who claim to be the nervous type have noted the tranquilizing effect of breastfeeding. Nursing can be a quieting and peaceful respite in the midst of noise, anxieties, and irritations. This is why some mothers will pick up their babies and nurse them on the rare night that they cannot sleep. Nursing, besides putting baby to sleep, can also put the mother to sleep. In addition, no matter how often or how long the baby nurses during the night, the mother is generally well rested, and this restfulness is truly a big bonus for the entire family. Mother can function better and enjoy her family more when she is not tired. Her good disposition makes for a smoothly running day. She, likewise, is not resentful — the baby did not keep her up all night, nor did her husband sleep through the night while she was up tending to the baby. In addition this practice eliminates a lot of decision making and possibly arguing between husband and wife. They do not have to decide who has to take care of the baby when he stirs or who will get up to warm the bottle. If the baby is already in their bed, the husband has another advantage — he doesn't have to get up even to bring the baby to bed. Indeed, the practice of the family bed can improve family life.

What about burping? Do you have to get up to burp your baby? Very frequently the baby who requires an occasional burping during the day may not require any burping at night. For a newborn who does require burping, it may help to remain in bed and place his head and shoulder area up over your stomach or to turn sideways and place him over your hip.

What about changing diapers? I used cloth cotton diapers folded to allow for extra absorbency during the night. A rubberized flannel square can be placed where the baby sleeps to protect the mattress in case of leakage. With breastfeeding, diaper rash is uncommon and a baby can usually go through the night without a change.

Mothers and fathers have told us how much they enjoy these night snuggles with their baby. Even dads like waking up with their child at their side. For working parents — whether it is the father or the mother — it is one time that the baby can stay in touch with mom or dad after having no contact with the parent during the day. I would strongly encourage working mothers to continue nursing so that 1) they can enjoy this special closeness with their baby and 2) they can easily care for their baby during the night without feeling fatigued in the morning.

Some parents ask whether this practice will interfere with intimacy between husband and wife. Not if you have any imagination. At times of intimacy it is not necessary to bring the baby to bed until afterwards when you are ready to sleep. Likewise, marital intimacies do not have to be confined to the bedroom.

Breastfeeding in bed has advantages for the baby too. This is one time when he can nurse to full contentment in quiet, cozy surroundings. This is a time when his mother won't be interrupted, a time when he can use the breast to fulfill his sucking needs. It is known that babies at times will nurse on and off for several hours while mother sleeps. This is common in the older breastfed child as well.

Another striking advantage is that the baby keeps in **touch** with mother in addition to his father. The baby has a critical need for bodily contact with his mother. He needs to be caressed, cuddled, held, or just carried about with his mother. Some psychologists and writers today are quite concerned that most babies receive very little contact with their mother. This physical closeness with mother is all too often lacking, especially in our American culture.

Ashley Montagu, in his book, *Touching: The Human Significance of the*

Skin,[8] demonstrates that the skin is the most important sensory organ we have and that the small child needs to receive much skin stimulation from his mother in order to survive physically and emotionally. The sense of touch on the skin is the most alert sense during sleep, and therefore he recommends sleeping with babies at least for the entire first and second year. If the mother objects to sleeping with her child during the second year, he advises the mother to lie with her child at bedtime until he falls asleep. He uses other cultures as an example of that type of "touch" mothering which is so lacking in the American culture. Sleeping with the child is characteristic of the mother in these cultures where the child has lots of skin-to-skin contact with mother and, of course, where breastfeeding is common. If this contact at bedtime is not provided, Montagu says a cuddly toy may help, but the child may resort to other activities, such as thumbsucking, rocking, and fondling of the genitals.

An historical article, "Of Babies, Beds and Teddy Bears" by Kenny and Schreiter,[9] provided us support in our learning years and documented the need for the infant to be in physical touch with his mother. The authors strongly encouraged sleeping with one's baby and supported this practice with psychological studies of other cultures. They showed how sleeping together was once an American tradition until twin beds became popular. Good mothering was defined as much holding and cuddling of the baby, with emphasis given to sleeping together at night.

Dr. William Sears points out the merits of the family bed and offers advice for problem sleep situations in his excellent books, *Nighttime Parenting*[10] and *SIDS*.[11] The medical, emotional and other advantages are demonstrated in his books. He clearly shows the benefits of co-sharing sleep, and I would recommend both of these books to any parent who has doubts about this practice.

I'm also convinced that nature's plan is easier for both baby and the parents. When parents step in to hurry the process along, it's more trouble than it is worth, and in most cases, the baby suffers and is not as happy. True, these babies can turn out to be wonderful human beings as grown children and adults, but why make things complicated and make more work for yourselves as parents when there is an easier way?

Natural child spacing

The mother who sleeps with her baby during the night is involved in a pattern of unrestricted breastfeeding. By taking care of the baby's needs for closeness, cuddling, and skin contact during the night, she also provides the opportunity for her baby to nurse as often as he pleases. In the Seventies a Chilean doctor confided to my husband that he encouraged mothers to cuddle their babies between their breasts during the night. This closeness stimulates the baby to nurse often and helps maintain the infertility of breastfeeding. This also happens when the baby is at the mother's side.

To show the influence of sleeping with the baby on the menstrual cycles, I would like to relate another true incident. The nursing mother experienced regular menstruation since childbirth. Her baby slept in another room, but that was to change when her husband went on a business trip for three months. When her husband left, she brought her nine-month-old baby to bed with her during the nights. She had no menstruation those three months during her husband's absence. The husband returned, her baby left her bed, and she soon noticed signs of returning fertility. I find this case extremely interesting since the only change in the nursing behavior during those three months of amenorrhea was the nursing that took place during the night while the baby slept with his mother.

Mothers should do the right things for the right reasons, so I don't recommend night feedings or other aspects of natural mothering *just* to prolong amenorrhea. They should come out of the mother's realization that the nighttime closeness and nursing are good for the baby and herself and that the extended amenorrhea is a natural side effect.

If this approach were taken generally, then there would be fewer mothers who complain that to experience breastfeeding's natural infertility they would have to set the alarm, get up a couple times during the night to get the baby, and so on. I sympathize with these mothers because they have knowingly or unknowingly adopted the practices of a Western culture that goes strongly against the natural practices of unrestricted nursing. It is difficult to achieve the natural side effects of breastfeeding when part of the natural relationship is thwarted. Perhaps the question these mothers — and dads too — should ask is, "If I were the baby, wouldn't I rather be close to my mother instead of all by myself? If I woke up during the night, wouldn't I rather be next to my mother who is ready to feed me rather than in a room with nobody else around?"

In the real world, we soon realize that we can't make it on our own. We need a friend, someone who will bear with us even when we are an inconvenience. So why not begin from the earliest months to let the baby know the friendship of his mother and his father? This is where the trust begins that is needed later for future relationships.

From everything said thus far, it should be evident that the mother who adopts this natural mothering approach isn't going to be thinking in terms of getting her baby to sleep through the night. She will let the baby set the pace. In fact, if the baby is an unusually heavy sleeper at first, she will want to encourage — not force — a nursing when she goes to bed and again when she first awakens. This relieves her breasts of excessive fullness and helps maintain a steady milk supply and avoid plugged ducts. It is also a most pleasant experience to nurse a sleepy baby at these times. The breast fullness seems to be nature's way of reminding the mother of her baby — and to be near her baby. It also helps the baby to get a regular intake of nourishment.

What if both you and your baby are such sound and long sleepers that your baby is not nursing at all during the night? The biological fact of life is that eight hours without nursing may cause an early return of fertility. But is there anything you can do when this occurs? Consider this: drink a large glass of water before you go to bed. After three to four hours, that may give you a bladder wake-up call. When you return to bed after your bathroom visit, put your sleeping baby to breast. He may well start to suckle.

In summary, if a baby wakes up at night because of a need that can be fulfilled at the breast, there is no easier and better way for the family to get back to sleep than by letting the baby nurse at his mother's side in bed. This not only helps to satisfy the baby's nutritional and emotional needs, but also satisfies the emotional needs of the mother. Not only is it restful for her, but she derives satisfaction in doing what is best for her baby and from having a contented and quiet baby as a result.

This Fourth Standard of sleeping with your baby during the night is crucial for maintaining normal breastfeeding infertility. Remember that research shows that the baby who sleeps with his mother will nurse three times more during the night than the baby who sleeps apart from his mother.

[1] Robert Lerer, "Babies' Sleep Habits Vary by Ethnic Background," *Journal News*, October 5, 1995.

[2] Lois Rogers, "Bed-Sharing May Cut Cot Deaths," *The Sunday Times*, October 8, 1995.

[3] Bill Manson, "Is Fatal Syndrome Halted When Babies Sleep With Mom?" *Washington Times*, December 26, 1993.

[4] Margaret Ribble, *The Rights of Infants*, New York: Columbia University Press, 1943, 1965.

[5] Lee Siegel, "Theory Links SIDS, Environment: Sleeping With Parents May Prevent Sudden Infant Death," *The Cincinnati Post*, May 28, 1985.

[6] James McKenna, S. Mosko, and R. Richard, "Bedsahring Promotes Breastfeeding," *Pediatrics*, 1997, 100(2), 214-19.

[7] *Pediatrics*, December 1997, 1035-39.

[8] Ashley Montagu, *Touching*, New York: Columbia University Press, 1971.

[9] James Kenny and Robert Schreiter, "Of Babies, Beds and Teddy Bears," *Marriage*, January 1971.

[10] William Sears, M.D., *Nighttime Parenting*, Schaumburg, Illinois: La Leche League Int., 1985.

[11] W. Sears, *SIDS*, Boston: Little, Brown and Co., 1995.

The Daily Nap

THE FIFTH STANDARD:
Sleep with your baby for a daily-nap feeding.

When we began our family in the 1960s, it was common for mothers to take the phone off the hook and take a nap with their children during the afternoon. There were no answering machines then! I find mothers today rarely take a nap with their little ones on a regular basis. Many mothers claim they are too busy, although I know a few homeschooling mothers who make taking a nap with their children a priority.

When I had a baby, a two-year-old, and a four-year-old, we all took a daily nap. If the oldest one was not tired, I would tell her to lie there quietly for a half-hour. If she was still awake after a half-hour, she could get up. Oftentimes she fell asleep before the half-hour was over. I knew I would get at least a half-hour of rest.

A daily nap refreshes a mother. She has more enthusiasm and a better disposition to finish the day. In addition, I believe that the daily nap with the baby may be extremely important for some mothers in maintaining amenorrhea. When we receive a call from a mother stating that she is doing natural mothering but has had an early return of menstruation, we now ask her, "Are you taking a daily nap with your baby?" The answer is almost always "no."

It must be emphasized here that taking a nap *does not mean* lying down to nurse the baby for his nap with the hope of getting up immediately to get things done as soon as the baby falls asleep. Taking a nap means the mother nurses, but she also takes a nap at the same time in order to get some extra, needed rest. The goal is a nap for mother as well as the baby with unrestricted nursing accomplished at the same time.

In the latter half of 1995 I analyzed the experiences of six mothers who had reported a return of menstruation from five weeks to four months post-partum while doing variations of ecological breastfeeding. One of these mothers did not respond to my additional questions. Four of the five early-return mothers who responded did not take a daily nap with their babies, and several did not do the family bed.

Four of the six mothers were tandem nursing which means they were nursing two children. Three of the four tandem-nursing mothers who responded did not take a daily nap with their baby; the fourth mother who tandem-nursed was the mother who did not respond. The three respondent tandem nursers believed that the extra nursing involved in nursing two children would be an additional help in maintaining amenorrhea.

The other two mothers who responded were nursing only one baby. One of these mothers had seven children, and with each one her menses returned at three to four months postpartum. Breastfeeding still gave her a spacing of 18 to 27 months between babies. She did not read this book, and she did not take daily naps with her babies.

The fifth respondent did take daily naps but had a surprising experience. She had her first menstrual period at five weeks postpartum and had regular periods after that. By eight weeks she discontinued her naps. She practiced the family bed, but her baby spent little time at the breast when the mother was awake. This baby completed a feeding in "5 to 10 minutes," was a contented baby, and "resisted any effort to get her to suckle longer." This mother and her husband wrote that as Christians they would never use contraception and began to chart her cycles. It wasn't until their baby was nine months old that they saw their first thermal shift. Ovulation had been suppressed until then.

I believe that those mothers who are nursing two babies need to avoid fatigue and need a nap even more than the mother who is nursing one baby. Fatigue can affect a woman's body, and I believe it can cause an early return of menstruation. In addition some experts believe that the natural child spacing mechanism works better when the mother is relaxed or when she is asleep.

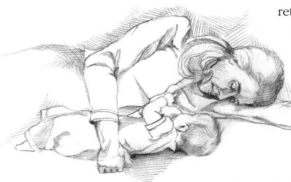

I experienced an early return (4½ months) with our fourth baby while getting this book ready for a publisher. Our breastfed baby was very alert, took brief naps, and did not sleep long in the evening until she retired with us. I used all my available time on the book, never took a nap, and simply did not get sufficient rest. The fatigue at that point in my life, I feel, was the reason for the early return of menstruation. Normal fertility, however, did not return until about 12 months postpartum, eight cycles later.

With continued frequent nursing day and night, especially with the use of the family bed, mothers who have an early return of menstruation often find that their fertility returns at a much later date. This is determined by temperature charting. On the other hand, nursing mothers who do not do the family bed, do not nurse frequently enough, or use pacifiers and bottles will usually have a quick return to fertility once menstruation returns prior to six months postpartum.

I'd like to stress that for some mothers who experience an early return of menstruation, not taking that daily nap could be a factor — as I now think it was for me. Naptime nursing and sleeping prevents fatigue; it also provides unrestricted nursing that produces strong hormonal surges in the mother's body at mid-day to help maintain amenorrhea after childbirth.

Nursing your baby during a nap is an important practice to consider if you would like the natural baby-spacing effect of breastfeeding — especially in our culture where many mothers work and a mother who naps may feel guilty about doing nothing. The unrestricted stimulation to the mother's breast from uninterrupted nursing during a daily nap may strongly influence her body chemistry toward natural infertility.

The Frequency Factor

SIXTH STANDARD:
Nurse frequently day and night, and avoid schedules.

Frequent and unrestricted nursing is a common occurrence among mothers who follow the ecological breastfeeding program described in this book. As I have mentioned before, it's this frequency which prolongs natural infertility following childbirth. In this chapter, I want to discuss two important conditions for frequent nursing — the absence of feeding schedules and the physical closeness of mother and baby. The oneness of the mother-baby relationship is crucial when following the ecological breastfeeding program and will be covered in the following chapter.

Frequent nursing

Since the first writing of this book in 1968, more attention has been given to frequent nursing episodes and their effect upon lactation amenorrhea. Dr. Peter Howie, working with a research team in Edinburgh, Scotland, asked why some nursing mothers ovulated much later than other nursing mothers. The answer was related to the frequency of suckling. Those nursing mothers who ovulated early nursed the least amount during the day, reduced the nursing times the fastest, introduced other foods quickly, and gave up the night feedings rapidly. On the other hand, Howie stated that the nursing mothers who ovulated later continued to give night feedings, nursed more often, introduced other foods slowly, and reduced their nursing times gradually. Howie concluded that "the effectiveness of suckling as an inhibitor of ovulation is certainly dependent upon breastfeeding practice. The resumption of ovulation may be dependent upon other factors as well, but certainly we would suggest that suckling is a major variable, if not *the* major variable in the control of postpartum ovulation and fertility." (Emphasis is in the original.)[1]

Howie and his associates centered their work on the introduction of solids and the absence of night feedings, practices they felt undermined the amount and frequency of suckling and led to the return of ovarian activity. A contemporary American study provided the same findings, that "night nursing after supplementation was a major factor in post-supplementation duration of amenorrhea."[2] In other words, among all nursing mothers who introduced other foods, the most important practice in delaying a return of their periods after supplementation was nursing during the night. More specifically, those mothers who introduced other foods later and who night-nursed for at least one hour once they started supplements remained in amenorrhea for six to ten months longer than those mothers who supplemented early and who reduced night feeds. As indicated in the previous chapter on night feedings, a night-nursing baby who sleeps with his mother nurses three times more than a nursing baby who sleeps in a separate room. Night-nursing for babies who sleep with their mothers is also a form of pacification, security, and physical reassurance during the night. And, most importantly, with this type of sleeping arrangement, there are no set schedules during the night.

The effects of the breastfeeding frequency factor upon fertility were also studied by James Wood, research scientist at the University of Michigan's Population Studies Center. His subjects were a New Guinea people, the Gainj, whose breastfeeding episodes are short and frequent. The child nurses on demand day and night, and he always sleeps with his mother. He begins solids at about nine to twelve months of age; complete weaning occurs at or near the child's third birthday. "The first solid foods given to the child (starchy tubers, bananas, papayas) are comparatively poor in nutrition so that breastmilk remains the only reliable source of high quality protein and fat in the child's diet well into the second or even third year of life."

The demographic picture demonstrates the spacing value of breastfeeding among this people who do not practice contraception or abortion. The researchers explained that if these Gainj women abandoned breastfeeding, they would reduce their average birth interval from 44 months to about 21 months, and the number of live births would more than double per woman from 4.3 to 9.2. As the researchers concluded, "the reproductive consequences of breastfeeding in this population are profound."

Dr. Wood and his team also recorded the frequency and intervals of the Gainj nursing sessions. With their infants, these women averaged 24-minute intervals; with their three-year-olds, they averaged about 80 minutes between nursings. The important thing is that the reduction in suckling frequency occurred very slowly. The research team concluded: "The finding that suckling frequency is high and changes only slowly over time appears to be of special importance in explaining the prolonged contraceptive effect of breastfeeding in this population."[3]

The !Kung tribe of Kalahari Desert in southern Africa has mothering and breastfeeding frequency patterns similar to those of the Gainj people. (The ! in !Kung represents a tongue clucking sound.) Researchers Konner and Worthman found that !Kung women were *conceiving* on the average of 35 months postpartum, thus allowing almost four years between the birth of their babies. They also observed that among this non-contracepting people the little one remained physically close to his mother day and night during the first two years. !Kung babies nurse several times each hour for just a few minutes each time. Konner and Worthman concluded that the frequency factor was the most likely key to the child spacing among this people.[4]

Nursing one's baby several times during the hour seems to be the norm, according to Dr. R. V. Short. He referred to two groups of hunter-gatherers: the !Kung tribe just mentioned and another tribe in Papua, New Guinea, where mothers also nurse frequently. He thinks that "the biochemical composition of human milk, which is low in fat, protein and dry matter" fits into the need for frequent suckling. While "this high frequency of suckling may seem abnormal at first," Dr. Short holds that is probably nature's norm. Even the chimps and the gorillas (the human species' closest relatives) suckle several times an hour in the wild, sleep with their babies, and have birth intervals of four or five years — similar to the two previously mentioned primitive tribes. Dr. Short credits the frequent suckling stimulus as "the crucial factor in causing the contraceptive effect" of breastfeeding.[5]

Do we get similar conclusions among American nursing mothers? American mothers are not accustomed to frequent nursing like the previously mentioned tribes. Dr. William Taylor has worked with Couple to Couple League mothers, a group that would be more inclined to follow more of the mothering practices typical of traditional breastfeeding cultures. The 72 American mothers in his study averaged 14 months of postpartum infertility. Dr. Taylor's research reaffirms past conclusions: what is important for breastfeeding infertility is short intervals between feedings. Those mothers who nursed the same amount of time per day but did so with long feedings and long intervals tended to ovulate earlier. The study also showed that those mothers who scheduled their nursing, introduced other liquids early, and left their baby alone at an early age also ovulated earlier.[6]

Avoid schedules

To do ecological breastfeeding, ignore advice about schedules — unless, of course, there is a serious medical reason for them. Someone will probably tell you that you will be feeding your baby at such-and-such-a time every day and that by a certain age you will be nursing only three or four times during the day. Someone else might tell you to nurse at least twenty minutes on each side or to nurse only five minutes on each side. One friend told me that she was told when she could bathe the baby, put it to sleep, and play with him! Obviously, such schedules are geared for adults and not for babies. Schedules don't focus on the true needs of a baby or his feelings — whether or not the baby is hungry or full, tired or sociable, dirty or clean.

The popular four-hour schedule is not popular with breastfed babies. Many breastfed babies will nurse several times during that amount of time. On occasion you may find yourself nursing your baby quite often, even within the same hour. Don't be surprised. After all, we adults often get up from the table only to find ourselves snacking an hour later or drinking between meals.

Some parents feel that a baby should be put on a schedule so he will not manipulate them. They fear that the baby will control the mother unless she controls him. Allegedly, he can even ruin family life and be a threat to a good marriage unless he is strictly scheduled and shown his place in the home! The emphasis here is on power rather than love. A baby has no complex ideas about controlling anyone. Nor can a baby and his needs be blamed for a deteriorating marital relationship. On the contrary, the sight of one's spouse going out of his or her way to take care of the baby's needs can be a source of renewed pride, but this is not to say that a baby is a cure for a poor marriage relationship. A baby has no plan for making people happy or unhappy.

Schedules simply have no place in natural mothering. In bottlefeeding, they serve the purpose of keeping babies from being starved by some mothers and overstuffed by others. However, in nature's baby care plan, mother and baby are always together, and the mother quickly senses her baby's nursing needs. This can contribute to your self-esteem as you realize your unique importance for your baby; it can also help develop your capacity for self-giving as you respond to his needs instead of scheduling him to fit your convenience.

Nursing mothers generally comment that things run more smoothly once they accept the more frequent feedings and forget the clock — and this applies even when the baby is older. In brief, rules are confusing because the schedule says one thing and the baby is telling mother something else. Mothering and breastfeeding are usually easier for both you and your baby when you take your cues from your baby and learn to relax with this flexibility and to simply enjoy him.

From the preceding paragraph it should be clear why schedules will most likely upset the breastfeeding baby-spacing ecology. The baby who is allowed to develop under the natural mothering program may be nursing every couple of hours during the day, sometimes even more frequently, and nursing during the night and during mother's nap. Thus the mother receives the frequent suckling stimulation that is necessary for her fertility to remain at rest.

Culture and attitude

Does this information change our thinking and help us to see frequent suckling as a normal occurrence — even a desirable goal? How often does it happen that a mother who severely limits suckling at the breast feels a need to supplement her milk or finds that her baby is not gaining well or appears to be hungry most of the time? Unfortunately, Western culture looks negatively upon frequent suckling and views a pattern of only three to five nursings a day as a desirable goal.

In our bottlefeeding society many American nursing mothers feel compelled to express milk in a bottle or use formula when they are away from home. I'm sure this practice is also common in other countries where bottlefeeding is unfortunately the "norm." Mothers have noticed a return of menstruation after visiting relatives over the holidays. They find themselves in an environment unfavorable towards breastfeeding, and they reduce their nursings considerably. Our society discourages public nursing, even *modest public nursing*, or nursing outside the family circle so that most people never see a baby at the breast. If they have seen a baby nurse, most likely the baby was their brother or sister or a very close relative's. I married at age 23, and up to that time I had never seen a mother nurse her baby.

If you want to do ecological breastfeeding with unrestricted nursing in a society where this type of breastfeeding is often unwelcome, you need determination. You can learn how to nurse modestly anywhere and to nurse comfortably in various social situations so you do not need to reduce your nursings. As your baby continues to nurse frequently with age, you will learn to be more comfortable with this continued pattern as well. The studies I have quoted reinforce what I have learned from personal experience and from other nursing mothers — namely, that with long-term nursing the frequency continues for an extended period of time and gradually diminishes toward the time of complete weaning. Usually the frequency of nursing is such that a mother hardly notices any changes in the frequency because the change is so gradual; but she may notice changes toward the end of the breastfeeding relationship.

It may sound as if all a mother does is nurse her baby and does nothing else. This is a false picture, although there are a few exceptions — especially during the early months. I have heard a few nursing mothers say their babies required constant nursing. This is unusual, though, and not the norm. With ecological breastfeeding, your baby nurses frequently but the feedings are brief. The long feedings usually occur when your baby is upset or hurt — which usually isn't often — and when he is tired prior to falling asleep. Some of these "tired" times are no inconvenience because you can also sleep when your baby is tired during your nap and during the night. You can reassure yourself from the research and the experience of other nursing mothers that your baby's frequent nursing pattern is normal, is part of God's plan for mother and baby with its many benefits, and is the type of breastfeeding and mothering associated with extended postpartum infertility.

[1] Peter Howie, "Synopsis of Research on Breastfeeding and Fertility," *Breastfeeding and Natural Family Planning*, Bethesda, Maryland: KM Associates, 1986.
[2] M. Elias, et al., "Nursing Practices and Lactation Amenorrhea," *Journal of Biosocial Science*, January 1986.
[3] J. Wood, "Lactation and Birth Spacing," *Journal of Biosocial Science*, Suppl., 9(1985), 159.

[4] M. Konner and C. Worthman, "Nursing Frequency, Gonadal Function, and Birth Spacing Among !Kung Hunter-Gatherers," *Science*, February 15, 1980, 788.

[5] R. Short, "Breast Feeding," *Scientific American*, April 1984, 35.

[6] W. Taylor, R. Smith, and S. Samuels, "Post-Partum Anovulation in Nursing Mothers," *Journal of Tropical Pediatrics*, December 1991, 286-292.

8

Mother and Baby As One

SEVENTH STANDARD:
Avoid any practice that restricts nursing or separates you from your baby.

Nature intends mother and baby to be one. In fact, a nursing mother who gives her total love and care to her baby will experience a relationship that she may never have with other persons. As one mother told me, "This is the first time I ever felt truly needed, that I was irreplaceable." Another mother said that her idea of heaven was to nurse a baby! This love relationship is built in naturally — the mother's body is geared toward giving by the continuous production of milk. Likewise, the production of milk provides her with a mothering hormone, prolactin, that helps her to feel more motherly. Nature has her own built-in laws for the child's development, and today her ways are being discovered more and more by researchers in the field and, unfortunately, are being ignored more and more by parents.

A chief ingredient for a healthy start in life is the presence of a continuous loving relationship with one mother figure. Nature has arranged this type of care through the oneness of mother and child through breastfeeding. Contrary to the opinion that you will spoil your baby by responding promptly to his needs, we are now being told that you can't give the baby too much love. Love him, enjoy him, meet his needs, and respond to his smiles, cries, and discomforts. Again, nature has already ensured that babies will receive this constant, individualized loving attention through the breastfeeding that only a mother can provide.

Fear of spoiling

Unfortunately some of our cultural theories concerning childcare lack common sense and feelings. Mothers are told that they should let their babies cry. After all, the theory goes, it is good for their lungs, or it is not good for the baby to control the parent. Some authors and doctors are quoted as saying that it is normal for babies to cry two to three hours a day. No! It is not normal for babies to cry for several hours a day. If a normal, healthy baby is crying that long daily, then this is usually a reflection of the parents' poor parenting skills, and the parents are the ones who need to change. The baby is often looked upon as a "thing" without feelings, almost lacking any human rights to be heard, understood, and loved. There are enough frustrations that occur naturally in everyday living without parents adding to them as a matter of policy.

All of this is done under the name of "not spoiling the baby." Spoiling a baby in this context refers to giving him attention of some kind when he cries or fusses or even when he is contented. It is feared that the baby is trying to get attention that he doesn't really need and is therefore being selfish. However, at his early age a baby's wants are simply the expression of basic human needs, both nutritional and emotional. A baby can't distinguish between legitimate needs and self-centered, unnecessary wants. When he fusses or cries, it is because he has a need that might very well be emotional rather than physical. Some writers have said that Mother Nature provided a built-in fussiness for babies so they will get some handling and comfort from their parents. I always felt that changing diapers was a blessing for many babies who do not get much attention from their mother. At least at these times the mother gives the baby a little bit of attention. Others have expressed concern about the "good" baby who is never picked up. The point is this: love demands that parents take care of their baby's needs, and you don't spoil a baby by taking care of his needs in a loving way. Natural mothering provides lots of personal contact with the baby, and it is eminently well suited for taking care of the baby's nutritional and emotional needs.

Leaving the baby

In a bottlefeeding culture baby-sitters are frequently used so mother can leave her baby. This is not very easy to do with the natural mothering program because the baby will need his mother for food at least within a couple of hours if not sooner. Some nursing mothers express their own milk to have on hand for the times they leave their baby. The same holds true for those dedicated nursing mothers who simply cannot avoid employment outside the home. However, ecological breastfeeding basically means that a mother remains with her baby. A mother who is interested in natural mothering and its related child spacing effect should desire this oneness that nature intended between mother and child. In fact she will soon discover that she does not desire to leave her baby; instead she makes every effort to be with her baby no matter where she goes.

Another common goal in a bottlefeeding society is to "be relieved of the baby." Thus leaving one's baby or children once or twice a week becomes a conscious goal for parents. Some justify their leaving by saying it is good for the baby to be exposed to a variety of people. The more people the baby is exposed to the better, so that the baby will be social from the beginning — so that theory goes. Others consider this separation necessary in order to keep one's sanity or to maintain a happy marriage.

A friend of ours expressed dismay when she learned we always included the children in our trips. She informed me critically that getting away by yourselves as a couple once or twice a year was necessary if you wanted to have a happy marriage. This is exactly what they did. Yet, sad to say, their marriage ended in divorce years later. Both John and I feel that the goal shouldn't be to get away from your children, especially when they are extremely young. Our first two children were about one and three years old when she offered me this advice. We feel the goal should be to maintain your closeness as a couple without leaving your children.

I might also add that my parents always included my sister and me on all trips and vacations. But my husband remembers being excluded from his parents' trips as a small boy, and this is one area where he wishes his parents had done it differently. So because of past experiences for both of us, leaving the children at home for vacations was not even a consideration.

It is becoming more popular for couples to vacation without their babies. Remember that babies have no concept of time. They have no idea where you are or when you will return. Parents, especially the mother, should have bonded to her baby. If so, the baby should miss her dearly. Usually the nursing intensifies the bonding. Imagine how you would feel if your spouse left one day and you did not hear from him at all for one or two weeks. You had no idea why he left nor did you know when he would return. Most of us in this situation would be concerned, upset, maybe mad, and hurt. That's similar to the feelings of a "deserted" baby.

Even older children can resent "temporary desertion." Some years ago after a day of children's tennis matches, a group of parents and children met to socialize over a meal. Sleeping became the topic. A young girl of about 12 years old said that she could not sleep unless her mother was near. In fact, she said she screams if she awakens in her room to find that her mother is not there. As a result her parents often let her sleep in a sleeping bag near their bed. I asked her mother if she had ever left her daughter for an extended period of time. The mother said "no." Then later in the evening the mother spoke of her trip to Australia so her husband could give a lecture tour. His talks were so well received that they went again. Of course, they left their daughter in the care of people she liked. But the daughter, hearing this, related how much she hated it.

This is not a book on homeschooling, but homeschooling parents can take a child — young or older — on a trip and make it an educational experience. When our youngest child was 15, we had an opportunity to spend eight full days in Rome; homeschooling made it possible to take our son with us.

With natural mothering, however, there are simply times when you cannot go with your husband on a business or social trip. There were two previous trips to Rome that my husband made when I could not go. No one seemed to understand why I stayed home. But my husband understood and was very supportive, even though being in Rome without his wife was definitely lonely for him.

In the Couple to Couple League we promote ecological breastfeeding and also encourage stay-at-home mothering, at least during the first three years of life. Some couples are not accepted in the teacher training program because the mother plans to work soon after the birth of a baby. Our Director of Teacher Training says it saddens him to hear from these mothers who are already planning to de-bond with their babies so they can leave them in the care of another person. Support for remaining one with your baby is a rarity in our culture. It is also cyclical: many young parents today had parents who worked, and they do not even consider doing it differently.

I know of one breastfed baby who went on a nursing strike when his mother went back to work for two full days a week. He would refuse to nurse by throwing his head back and away from the breast. She soon decided to remain home because this was best for her baby. The baby soon rejected any bottle filled with breastmilk, even from his loving father. This baby is blessed because his parents love him dearly and listen to his needs. They are now taking him to parties and events they would have never considered doing during the pregnancy or when their baby was a newborn. The strong bonds of breastfeeding help parents to grow, and future plans of the parents can be changed as a result of that bonding.

Oneness brings enjoyment

Do mothers involved in natural mothering need a break from their babies? Let's listen to Dr. Thomas Lambo who described the mothering customs of the African mother in an interview for *Psychology Today*.[1] This psychiatrist said that the traditional African mother is inseparable from her child during its first 15 months after birth. The mother meets her child's needs freely and even anticipates them before the child begins to whimper. Gradually, the child is given over to other members of the family who continue to give the child physical affection. Thus the child grows up in a secure environment of love and approval. The interviewer was interested in knowing if the African mother became irritated or annoyed with her child as a result of being with him continuously. Dr. Lambo said that, unlike women elsewhere in Western cultures, the African mother exhibits very warm and affectionate feelings toward her baby and that breastfeeding plays a part in the mothering relationship. With increased urbanization, Dr. Lambo is concerned that this mothering pattern might be changed in Africa. He stated that when women become involved in two roles, the traditional mother-infant relationship of inseparability undergoes a drastic change, and he is worried that this method of childcare may be affected or lost to the African people. This article showed several things: that mothers can **enjoy** this oneness with their babies, that closeness and inseparability might play a big factor in this enjoyment, and that breastfeeding produces the environment for such closeness.

Mother-baby togetherness is a practice that usually produces happy mothers and happy babies. When asked why her baby is so good, a typical ecological breastfeeding mom tells people that it's because he goes everywhere with her. The mother's presence is what makes the baby so content!

Mothers who practice ecological breastfeeding discover they want to be with their babies. Usually in our society mothers enjoy a break away from the baby, so they can do other things. Not true for the mother who nurses her baby often. Being away from her baby is a painful, unpleasant experience, and she promises to avoid future separations. The mother enjoys her baby and keeps him with her.

One mother wrote: "He comes with me everywhere. I enjoy taking him with me. I could not leave him as it would be like amputating a limb and leaving it behind."

Sometimes the pleasantness of mother-baby togetherness is contagious, as another mother relates:

> I nursed my first baby for 4½ months (three months exlusively), but considered it a nursing failure. The baby did not gain well on breastfeeding alone as I used schedules and no lying-down nursing. Our second was nursed frequently — about every two hours for the first year, slept with us, and went everywhere with us (including conventions, weddings, parties, meetings, and restaurants). Our emotional bond is much different and I really enjoyed this baby. As a result of our example, at least three of our friends with previously bottlefed, baby-sat babies are now following natural mothering and loving it. Having our happy, well-behaved baby with us all the time has been a joy, and many people have remarked on this.

Carrying

When a mother brings baby with her, her baby is usually soothed and comforted by being carried close to her. I have come to believe that God meant for mothers to hold their babies a lot! Some experts say that babies have a high need to be near their mother and that this need is as important as their need for nutrition — and may be even more important. Inseparability facilitates frequent nursing and tends to prolong breastfeeding. Susan Dillman explains well this association of carrying and frequent nursing:

> Species whose mothers leave their babies have milk that is high in protein and fat and they space their feedings from every two to fifteen hours. However, those mammals that stay with their young secrete milk which is low in protein and fat and they feed their babies almost continually. Human milk is low in fat and extremely low in protein, suggesting that the human infant is adapted to frequent feeding and extensive maternal contact. Because babies are unable to follow their mothers around at birth and we don't spend months hibernating with them, scientists have identified the human pattern of infant care as that of carrying.[2]

Carrying also means a contented baby, with crying being an unusual occurrence. In other countries where inseparability is practiced, crying is not observed. Yet, as Maria Montessori points out, "crying of children is a problem in Western countries," and parents often "discuss what to do to quiet the baby and how to keep him happy." She claims the child is mentally bored and "the only remedy is to release him from solitude and let him join in social life." Montessori explains in great length the many carrying devices women have used to carry a baby on their bodies, and she also shows how the baby learns in a variety of ways when the mother shares her life with her child.[3]

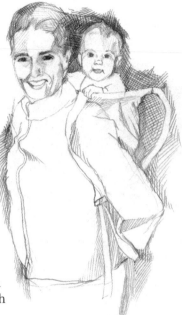

Some mothers take this inseparability practice very seriously. A group of mothers in Arizona were followers of Dr. James Clark Moloney and his views on "marsupial mothering." This former professor of psychiatry had written many articles on mother-baby "physical" togetherness. Having been exposed to his views, these mothers carried their babies on their person from birth on. Dr. Moloney felt that marsupial mothering should last for ten months or more, that babies thrive with an available, responsive, and loving mother, and that carrying or marsupial mothering was the best approach. His concern with the American mother was that many of them avoided such intimacy with their babies.

Some mothers have a small child who seems to need his mother all the time. The following letter shows that good things happen when a mother tries to meet those needs generously:

> My fourth child had an unusually intense need for my physical presence. His need to have me available to meet his needs was very intense and long-lasting. He was so possessive of my attention that I really felt I ended up neglecting my other children (let us not even consider the housework!). I had to pour everything I had into meeting his needs.
>
> This baby would not let me out of his sight. I tried to leave him with his father from time to time, but was unable to do so until he was 18 months of age. He either went with me or I didn't go. I was glad that I had three other more normal children because this baby was constantly on my body for the first 18 months of life. I used a Gerry carrier exclusively. I really needed the support my La Leche League group offered me, even though I knew I was doing the right thing by meeting all his needs. We left him with his grandmother about two times a year until he was two.
>
> All the rest of society told me there was something wrong with me to produce such a dependent child, and there was something wrong with him for being that way. In brave moments I would just laugh and tell them that I expected great things from Joe, that the love you invest in children is re-

turned to you and the world a thousandfold when they mature, and I had poured more love into Joe than any other child on earth. Joe reached the independence of the average 18-month-old when he turned three. We debated about sending him to school when he came of age. Obviously he was unable to stand the separation of school during the pre-school years. When he turned six, he reached another new level of independence and started the first grade the very next month very happily.

At the time of this writing, Joe is seven years old, and quite the most self-assured, independent, loving, thoughtful child you have ever seen. I know God has a plan for Joe. I'm glad I met his needs when he was a baby.

I never could have done so without the support of *Breastfeeding and Natural Child Spacing*. I feel confident that if I had been unwilling or unable to meet his needs he would have been a very different person, equally as angry and evil as he now is happy and good. Thanks from all of us.

This story may offer encouragement to those mothers who have a similar high-need baby or to the mother who has several days where the baby seems to make excessive demands. A few mothers who felt their older baby or child was too clingy have mentioned later that much of the problem stemmed from their own attitude, that they did not accept their child's needs at an older age. Once their attitude changed, they soon discovered that their child's behavior also changed for the better.

Babies, even older babies, feel secure in mom's loving presence. The feeding embrace tells a little one that he is loved and very special, and the baby who has a mother who is readily available does not feel threatened by separation. This leads us to another advantage of inseparability: some breastfeeding problems are usually absent.

The absence of some problems

Some mothers have written that their babies cry when they are put in a crib after being nursed to sleep. Some claim that their babies cry whenever they leave the room. Some notice that their babies cry upon awakening because they find that mother is not there. As one mother said about her baby: "When she realizes she's alone, she starts to cry." These situations are usually eliminated with mother-baby togetherness. The baby feels the closeness of mother's presence and does not fear that mother is trying to leave him. The baby is always with his mother. Very simply, where mother goes, the baby goes. And where mother is, baby is. The baby who is always in close proximity to his mother is a very secure baby.

A homeschooling, breastfeeding mother called me for help. Her baby screamed whenever she tried to put him in his crib. It soon became clear that she was isolating the baby in his crib so that she could homeschool her other children. I pointed out the advantage of breastfeeding, that this could be done while she homeschooled and that the baby could remain near her whether awake or asleep. I even mentioned a close friend who homeschools on her couch so that she is readily available to a nursing baby or toddler. I called her one week later. Guess where the baby was when I called? On her person in a carrier and things were much better!

Granted, it is much easier to "see" breastmilk when breastfeeding. We know the baby needs that food. On the other hand, we do not "see" the need for nurturing. It's intangible. And many mothers today do not believe that they are that important to their babies. After all, we are constantly being told that anyone can replace us. But that's a lie. A mother is simply irreplaceable.

In our society this "togetherness" practice takes some readjustment in thinking. I know it did for me. I went from "Where am I going and who will I leave the baby with?" to trying to leave only when the baby was asleep and returning when necessary for a nursing. The final change came when I took the baby or toddler or small child with me everywhere, no matter what others thought.

The same philosophy can be applied at home. Running downstairs to do the laundry or upstairs to make a bed does not have to separate you from your child. You simply bring him with you. When the small one falls asleep (usually nursing to sleep), keep the sleeping child right in the area where you will be. This means that the child is not sleeping in his crib in a room separated from mom's activity or in a room secluded upstairs away from the household activity.

This idea of having the baby or little one sleeping near where the mother is may seem far-fetched, but in practice it is so convenient. I used a firm quilt placed on the floor in the corner or away from the flow of traffic. If it was hot, there was no need for covering the baby. If it was cold, I dressed them accordingly or covered them with appropriate covers. It was easy and convenient to lie down and nurse the child to sleep. I often got a short rest at this time. After the child had fallen asleep, I could easily get up without interfering with the child's sleep. When the child awoke, I was readily available.

Mothers and fathers also have to realize that babies do not sleep all the time. Sometimes a baby takes only half-hour naps, sometimes an hour, and sometimes two hours. But soon they will probably be awake more during the daytime than asleep. A small infant who's awake can be carried around on his mother's body or he can be placed on the floor near where his mother is working.

In the early or late evening, an infant or older baby can be nursed to sleep in the rocking chair and then placed near mom and dad on the floor. This is a convenient time for the couple to share their day with each other or their various thoughts or preoccupations. A couple who desire sexual relations that evening can let the baby sleep nearby and later bring the baby to bed with them.

Even a pre-schooler enjoys mother's presence while falling asleep at night. Dad may also be an acceptable substitute as the child grows in age.

This time is a great way to end the day and to make the child feel good about himself if things did not go well that day. The time can be used for quiet reading, singing, praying and storytelling.

Natural child spacing

The practice of mother-baby togetherness also has an impact on natural child spacing. The following example helps to make this point. In a study conducted in the West African country of Rwanda, it was discovered that there were no differences in the birth intervals of bottlefeeding mothers in the city compared to those in the rural areas. On the other hand, among breastfeeding mothers, there were significant differences. The city mothers were already developing patterns of separation from their babies; 75% of the city breastfeeding mothers *conceived* between 6 and 15 months postpartum. However, in the rural areas, mothers still kept their babies with them all the time; 75% of the rural breastfeeding mothers *conceived* between 24 and 29 months postpartum. In this culture there were no contraceptives used or taboos against intercourse after childbirth. The researchers concluded that the only difference they could see between the two breastfeeding groups was the amount of physical contact the baby had with his mother.[4]

In summary, inseparability is the key to ecological breastfeeding. A mother has to be available to meet her baby's needs. This closeness is the basis for the other standards of ecological breastfeeding. For example, frequent and unrestricted nursing — day and night — is a natural consequence of this togetherness. The result is prolonged postpartum infertility and, most importantly, happier mothers and babies.

[1] James Breetveld, "A Brief Conversation with Thomas Lambo," *Psychology Today*, February 1972, 63-65.
[2] S. Dillman, "A Call to Arms," *Mothering*, Winter 1985, 92.
[3] Maria Montesorri, *The Absorbent Mind*, New York: Dell, 1967, 107.
[4] M. Bonte et al., "Influence of the Socio-Economic Level on the Conception Rate During Lactation," *Int. Journal of Fertility*, 19(1974), 97-102.

Weaning and the Return of Fertility

Natural weaning

There are three points to consider about natural weaning. First, weaning is a process that begins as soon as the baby starts taking anything other than his mother's milk at the breast. Second, weaning, in this sense, can last for several years. Third, with extended ecological breastfeeding there are, on the average, more months of postpartum infertility after "weaning" starts than during the months of exclusive breastfeeding.

The time will come when your baby begins to wean himself from nutritional dependence at your breasts to the stage where he is completely independent of your body as a food source. The mother who desires the most natural weaning of her baby and the benefits of natural child spacing has to realize that there are different methods of weaning and that only one of these is quite conducive to natural child spacing.

In many quarters there is the practice of weaning a baby or toddler abruptly. Such a form of weaning completely terminates any child-spacing effect that had been derived from breastfeeding and that might be continued for some time in a more gradual weaning process. On the other hand, the natural means of weaning that can prolong the child-spacing effect of breastfeeding is a very gradual process that is controlled largely by the baby himself. Gradual weaning at the right time can extend breastfeeding infertility considerably.

There are two key factors in what I call natural weaning. First, mother has to wait until the baby is **ready** for solids; secondly, she has to wean her baby **gradually** off the breast at her child's pace. Early weaning — by which I mean not only hasty weaning but the early use of solids, bottles, or cups — may be gradual, but it is not what I call **natural** weaning. Nature apparently intended that the baby receive only milk from its mother in the first months of life. Any deviation from this natural plan, such as early weaning, usually brings with it a short history of breastfeeding. Early weaning or short-term cultural nursing usually means an early return of fertility after childbirth.

When natural weaning occurs, some babies may wean themselves rather quickly. Others will continue to nurse quite heavily for a long period of time even though they are eating many solid foods. **An older baby of**

increasing size, activity, and appetite may begin to take other food and still continue to nurse as much as before. Frequent nursing may continue well into the second or third year of life. Since frequent or unrestricted nursing is the major factor in breastfeeding infertility, you can see how gradual, natural weaning can extend postpartum infertility.

If the baby is to set the pace, how can you tell when your baby is ready for his first taste of solid food? The answer is simple — your baby's actions will tell you when he is ready. A baby has an early desire to put everything into his mouth. There will come a time when the older baby, sitting on your lap at the table, will not be satisfied until he can have some of the food he sees in front of him. Or he will start to feed himself with his fingers when he is ready. The same holds true for the cup. Someday he will want a cup and will make his new desires quite evident. In other words, you don't need to spoon-feed a child or offer a cup in an effort to introduce baby to his first solid food or liquids. Just wait and let your baby call the shots.

Some mothers want some specific guidelines concerning starting other foods. My suggestion is to follow the American Academy of Pediatrics' strong recommendations of exclusive breastfeeding for the first six months of life. In other words, simply enjoy your baby and do exclusive breast-feeding during his first six months of life. After that, gradually introduce solids when your baby is interested. Normally, a baby begins to show an interest in solids between six and nine months of life. Our children who were involved with ecological breastfeeding showed an interest in other foods at about eight months of age. They also began slowly by taking little bits at a time.

A mother may offer mashed banana or a smashed pea to her six month old baby only to find the baby refusing it. The mother can then wait for several weeks before trying again. Although some mothers have been taught by society that it is "good" for the baby to eat lots of food three times a day right from the start, nature generally sets a slower pace.

Once her baby shows an interest in food, the nursing mother can still be flexible about her baby's needs. Just as there was no rigid feeding schedule while completely nursing, so there will be no rigid feeding schedule during the weaning phase of breastfeeding. She may offer him a little food once or twice a day; another day she may be surprised to find that her baby only nursed the entire day. Gradually, however, he will be at the table for most of the family meals.

Up to now, the nursing mother has not had the mess of spoon-feeding a young infant nor the problem of cleaning bibs or stained shirts. She will find now that feeding solids to an older baby is very easy. At the table the mother can mash the food with a fork, and some foods, such as fresh fruit, can be scraped with a spoon. Older babies can pick up certain foods that can be cut in thin strips. The mother should avoid giving her baby sweet foods of the candy and cookie variety. She also should avoid excess use of filler foods such as processed white bread and crackers. These foods may decrease her baby's desire to eat good foods, and they may be harmful to his teeth. Note well: by using your own table foods, you can avoid the costs of buying prepared "baby foods." With our first baby, we bought a few jars of baby food when we were camping; she did not like this canned food. With our last four children, we did not buy a single jar of baby food.

It should be remembered that the beginning of solid food does not mean an end to breastfeeding: **solids at first are only a supplement to breastfeeding and not a replacement**. Nursings will still be periodic and frequent, if your baby desires them, day or night. Your baby may still want to nurse during the night or upon awakening in the morning. He may want to nurse at the table during or after a meal. Here's a good idea: in order to maintain a good milk supply, nurse prior to a "solids" feeding, especially during the first stages of introducing other foods. Continue to offer the breast as needed, and remember that your baby will most likely still want to be nursed to sleep. Breastmilk continues to be a nutritious food for the older baby or toddler and will continue to be his main liquid diet for many more months. Even after he shows an interest in a cup, he will most likely continue to nurse during the day and night.

Babies will wean themselves off the breast naturally. Unfortunately very few babies in our society wean naturally; their parents force the weaning process. A few babies will finish weaning naturally before their first birth-day, but this is early and rare. Most babies wean before or after their sec-ond, third, fourth, and, yes, even their fifth birthday. Three of my children nursed from four to five years. Many people are upset to hear that a one-year-old is still nursing, but think nothing of a two-year-old with a bottle in his hand. Thus, when someone expresses surprise at a baby still breastfeed-ing past his second or third birthday, the nursing mother might politely ask her friend if she would be surprised if the baby had an occasional bottle or used a pacifier at that age. Remember that toward the end of the weaning period your child will not nurse every few hours but may nurse only occa-sionally during the day — for example, before naps or during the night. The feedings before naps or bedtime are often the last feedings to be dropped.

There are a few other points I want to mention with respect to natural weaning. First, it would be wrong for a mother to withhold solids at her baby's expense. She should not consider prolonged 100% breastfeeding in order to prolong the absence of menstruation for a longer period when her baby really wants and needs solid foods. Secondly, natural weaning does not mean that she holds her baby back. A mother can't help but offer her baby encouragement over his progress. On the other hand, she will also realize that this slightly older child is still a baby in many ways and still needs to nurse. Just as she won't hold him back in order to prolong breast-feeding infertility, she also won't deprive him of his nursing in order to achieve another pregnancy. She learns to accept this "nursing" need of his approvingly and learns to enjoy this long-term relationship.

Birthdays are often a time for weaning. A mother may ask her child, for example, at his third birthday, "Are you ready to quit nursing now that you are three years old?" The child insists he still needs to nurse; he may cry at the thought of not nursing anymore. Then the mother can say, "Are you going to quit on your next birthday when you're four years old?" This sounds more distant and the child thinks that might be a good idea. Our last two children were not ready at their fourth birthday, but they both agreed they would be ready when they were five years old. I let the subject drop for an entire year. Then at the time of their fifth birthday, I asked each again. Both decided at this time that they were big enough to quit. And that was it. No effort on my part and no tears on their part.

Adult members on both sides of our family had severe allergy problems when they were young. My husband and my sister suffered greatly due to allergies during their childhood. Our children have been spared such suffering and I'm convinced it's not coincidental. I believe that long-term breast-feeding protected our children, especially one child who I am sure could have had severe problems if she had not been breastfed for five years.

It is hard to imagine a woman nursing a two-year-old or a four-year-old. These children look so big. I have known women who have nursed children who are even older than five years old. Although I have had the experience of nursing an older child, I still think to myself when I see a three or four year old that they're too big to be nursing. What I am trying to say is that it is different when it's **your** child. Also, that child is usually nursing only at home or only among close family members or friends.

Besides the health or physiological benefits, such as allergy prevention or reduction, there are many emotional or psychological reasons to continue the nursing. The closeness of the nurturing relationship makes discipline so easy by loving example and the child is so eager to please his mother to whom he is closely attached. Also the child feels he is loved and very special when the mother accepts the long-term breastfeeding relationship. The child also learns in an easy fashion through the language and conversations of his mother and by accompanying her wherever she goes.

It's sad that many mothers quit nursing during the early months because the experience of nursing an older child becomes even richer and fuller. Mothers have found the practice of baby-led weaning to be very satisfying as indicated by the following examples.

"Our two-year-old weaned himself recently. The first time he quit for a month. Then he resumed for another month and now he has given it up again. I'm glad he did the deciding. It really makes me feel right inside. I know you know the joys of nursing a toddler, but this is the first time for me and it was so rewarding, so special. I do think God was very wise in his plan for babies and mothers. I'm wondering if perhaps the nursing experience doesn't help the weaning that must come when the young adult leaves home."

"My youngest is now four years old and weaned about a week before his fourth birthday. He still has a little try once in a while but informs me I'm empty. I have enjoyed baby-led weaning so much and can see all the advantages so clearly. I only wish I'd been doing this with the first two, although they are reaping the benefits too. I can't think of anything that's more enjoyable and rewarding than being a mother."

"Nursing an older baby seemed to be a particular experience with me as Lennie didn't wean until she was three. Now my arms are so empty. I find much joy in the children as they are growing and maturing, but there is just that special **something** about breastfeeding that we don't ever experience again."

Return of menstruation

During the natural course of breastfeeding, a mother will eventually experience the return of menstruation, for during the weaning process the baby will gradually be taking less and less from the breast. The reduced frequency of nursings is probably the major factor in the return of menstruation and fertility even though the baby may still be receiving a good quantity of breastmilk. If the weaning process is a natural affair, the return of menstruation will usually occur while the mother is nursing her baby. If the weaning is abrupt, the return of menstruation normally occurs several weeks (two to eight) after the nursing has stopped. Any sort of weaning brings with it sooner or later the eventual return of menstruation.

The return of menstruation is generally a strong indicator of the future return of fertility. I say "future return" because ovulation usually does not occur before the first period following childbirth. Many nursing mothers have relied successfully on breastfeeding infertility during amenorrhea, and many mothers experience one to three infertile cycles after the return of menstruation. About 6% of nursing mothers who have babies six months or older will become pregnant before their first period, assuming regular intercourse and no fertility awareness or periodic abstinence. If mothers want additional spacing other than what the breastfeeding gives them, they can learn their fertility signs and switch to *systematic* natural family planning if a pregnancy is not desired. I refer interested readers to the "Natural Family Planning" chapter later in this book.

The absence of menstruation, especially during the first six months, provides a sense of security for the nursing mother who would like to avoid pregnancy soon after childbirth. This feeling of security can be lost if any bleeding or spotting occurs during the third, fourth, fifth, or sixth month postpartum. Some mothers experience spotting or bleeding in the early months, but then increase the nursings to hold back menstruation once again.

Spotting may also be a warning that menstruation or ovulation is around the corner. Indeed, a few mothers have conceived after spotting and without having had a regular menstruation. If a mother experiences pre-menstrual feelings during these early months, she might re-evaluate her schedule and aim for more rest and nursing. I had these feelings once and made a special effort to rest more at naptime and also during the night, and I let the baby nurse often during those rest times. The pre-menstrual feelings left and there was no menstruation.

Nursing mothers whose menstrual periods have not returned may be confused when they experience bleeding that is not menstrual in nature. The bleeding can be due to other factors. One mother had a Pap smear taken which resulted in some bleeding. She did not expect her periods to return until the baby was about a year old. The bleeding stopped and her periods did not return for months. Another friend had cauterization treatments for cervical erosion. She bled seven days after the first treatment and twenty days after the second treatment. This was confusing to the mother who wondered if the bleeding was due to menses or to the doctor's treatment. Maybe mothers could ask if such treatments have to be done now or if it would be possible to delay it for a year.

A group of nursing mothers in our community some years ago discussed the fact that while they had all experienced an absence of periods due to breastfeeding with previous babies, they were surprised with their present baby to have experienced a bleeding episode at about six weeks postpartum. These mothers wondered what caused this bleeding since their menstrual cycles did not resume and they went on to experience amenorrhea as they had done with previous babies. Some of the women felt the bleeding was caused by the resumption of coitus; others felt it might be due to increased activity around the time of bleeding. Some thought their body had not healed completely from the pregnancy and thus the bleeding occurred. We now know that it was probably due to changing hormones in the woman's body.

La Leche League shed new light on this in its 1981 revised manual, calling this six weeks bloody discharge not a true period but a "withdrawal bleeding" due to changing hormones. This issue was also addressed by an international group of doctors who met to discuss the conception rates of breastfeeding mothers. Their conclusions are called the Bellagio Consensus since they met in Bellagio, Italy in 1988. For the fully or nearly fully breastfeeding mother, they said, any vaginal bleeding up to the 56th day can be ignored. "Fully" would mean exclusive breastfeeding. After the 56th day, the nursing mother must 1) be fully or nearly fully breastfeeding and 2) remain in amenorrhea in order to enjoy a 98% rate of infertility during the first six months postpartum. Once either one is absent, the chance of pregnancy increases.[1] A mother who is truly practicing the full ecological breastfeeding/natural mothering program described in this book therefore has no reason to worry about bleeding up to 6 to 8 weeks postpartum. If an exclusively breastfeeding mother has menstrual bleeding after the 56th day postpartum, she can begin to chart her fertility signs and use systematic natural family planning while she continues to nurse.

The return of fertility does not mean an end to nursing. A mother can continue to nurse her baby or child while having menstrual cycles and even while pregnant. Nursing two children who are siblings is called tandem nursing and has been done for centuries. Weaning can occur during pregnancy. The mother may react negatively to nursing due to hormonal changes even though she had planned to nurse throughout the pregnancy. She may suddenly find nursing very painful. Some mothers may nurse during the discomfort. I found myself in this situation when one of our children was four years old. The nursing was so painful she did not want to hurt me and agreed to just a minute of nursing. Then, she said, back rubs would be sufficient. Other children may wean because the milk tastes different or is reduced in quantity. One of our godchildren was recently disappointed to find that his pregnant mother had no more milk. She assured him that there would be plenty when the baby came and he could have some then. He then decided that the baby would have one side and he would have the other!

Some mothers continue to satisfy the child's needs at the breast while pregnant and continue to nurse both the baby and other child after childbirth. This is especially true in other cultures where prolonged lactation is common. Several mothers have liked continued nursing because the older child did not resent the new baby. One mother wrote of her older nursing child:

> Her complete acceptance of nursing as a fact of life for herself and for the baby is as delightful and useful a thing as amenorrhea — in that jealousy in its usual forms with the birth of a new baby has been minimal; any reaction has been more like intrigued attention at odd moments. That's been particularly refreshing to me since our first early-weaned child was a most unhappy soul for ages when faced with a similar situation. So not only did I enjoy a completely successful two-year spacing between children but also this added bonus of a happy displaced toddler.

A mother nursing when pregnant should consider the consequences of her actions. Is her child ready for reduced nursings? Do other activities with mother suffice in place of a nursing? Many nursing children, even the older ones, will not be ready to wean; and, if so, there is really no reason to quit, assuming it is not painful to the mother. Actually, as we have seen from the above example, forced weaning may be most unpleasant after the birth of the newborn, whereas continued nursing may be advantageous under the circumstances. In addition, a child who has had his needs fully met by his mother and who knows his mother will continue to satisfy his needs and love him will be less inclined to be jealous; he has a secure relationship with his mother and the new baby does not pose any threat to his security. He is also more inclined to be concerned that the baby gets his needs met too. There is nothing more touching than to see a still-young brother or sister be upset at the first cry of the new baby and insist that Mommy take care of the baby right away.

I have also received a few letters from mothers who quit nursing during pregnancy because they felt they should but later were upset to learn that they could have continued the nursing. One such mother, who had a still-born, regretted her weaning decision during early pregnancy. A mother likewise may wean and later experience a miscarriage. Breastfeeding will not affect a good pregnancy, but adverse situations do happen whether one is nursing or not, and thus these possibilities are worth considering when making a decision. On the other hand, these considerations should not lead a mother to feel forced to continued nursing during pregnancy. She should feel free to do what she sees as best, everything considered.

Menstrual variation among mothers

Why does one mother nurse her completely breastfed baby and have periods while another mother introduces juices early and still does not experience a menstrual period? Why does one mother whose baby uses a pacifier regularly not experience a period until her nursing baby is two years old while another mother follows all the rules for natural mothering and experiences a period when her child is five months old? Apparently the amount of mothering and stimulation required at the breast to hold back menstruation varies among mothers, some of whom require more stimulation than others.

There is some evidence that the older a woman is and the more children she has had, the longer it will be before menstruation returns. However, this increase in amenorrhea is so small that one wonders if the experience built up over the years creates more confidence and, as a result, mothers nurse better and longer with each child. Better and longer lactation would tend to postpone menstruation a little longer. On the other hand, a few mothers have reported an earlier return of menstruation with advancing age. Maybe they are busier with more children and do not take the time to nurse as much or to get that daily nap. Some of these mothers have nursed other babies, yet with their new baby they are disappointed when menstruation returns earlier than ever before. A few mothers who were following the guidelines in this book have told me this has happened to them.

Likewise, babies vary. Each baby has different sucking and weaning needs. Some babies desire the breast more often than others. These factors are individual variations over which we have little control. However, they appear to be minor considerations for most mothers.

The most important considerations are those over which we have a great deal of control. Are we going to care for our babies at the breast naturally, or are we going to nurse but also offer breast substitutes? Are we going to sleep with our baby during the night? Are we going to take a daily nap with our nursing baby? Are we going to follow the complete ecological breastfeeding program? These decisions will make the most difference to the individual mother.

Here is one example that demonstrates how parenting choices can impact the return of fertility. This particular mother used only breastfeeding to space her babies. She nursed her first baby for 11 months and exclusively breastfed for the first five months. She gave night feedings for eight months and offered a pacifier frequently; her menstruation returned at six months postpartum and conception occurred at 12 months postpartum. With the second baby the mother nursed and slept with her baby for 26 months. Solids were offered at six months, but the baby did not take them until seven or eight months of age. This baby never had a pacifier and was given night feedings until 26 months old. Menstruation returned at 24 months and conception occurred at 25 months postpartum. As we see here, a change in mothering practices can affect the duration of amenorrhea and infertility for an individual mother.

For many mothers the mechanism involved is a very delicate one. Any decrease in the nursing may cause a return of menstruation. Eliminating one rule or practice from the Standards of ecological breastfeeding may shorten or eliminate any natural spacing effect for a particular woman. These mothers require lots of frequent and unrestricted nursing to hold back menstruation. Mothers who do exclusive breastfeeding and who experience an early return of fertility or menstruation are usually — but not always — not following the natural mothering program. One mother, for example, stated that she was exclusively breastfeeding and nursing her baby "all the time" when her periods returned. Upon further discussion with her, I learned that this mother fed the baby only during the day and then only once every four hours. Her baby was already sleeping through the night. After her periods return, the mother who requires lots of nursing stimulation will probably find that she will continue having regular periods even though the baby may increase his nursing at the breast.

On the other side of the coin, there are mothers who require very little stimulation to hold back menstruation. They can be down to several nursings a day and still not experience a return of menstruation. In addition, once their periods do resume, a little bit of increased nursing at the breast may influence their cycles. Increased nursing prior to ovulation may delay ovulation and thus the cycle would be longer than usual. Increased nursing after ovulation has occurred will not prolong the cycle. Delayed ovulation from increased nursing is more likely to occur during the first year after childbirth and is less likely to occur as the baby gets older.

The natural return of menstruation via natural mothering tends to provide more regularity for the nursing mother. Cultural nursing, with its use of artifacts as mother substitutes, usually results in a fairly early return of menstruation. For various reasons, including the variations in the young baby's suckling pattern, delayed ovulation and irregular cycles appear to be more commonly associated with an early return of menstruation than with a later return.

Average return of first menstruation

Generally speaking, when can you expect fertility to return? Our research shows that women who adopt the ecological breastfeeding program will **average** 14.5 months without periods following childbirth.[2] This is only an average. Some, an exceptional few, will experience a return before six months postpartum. Others will go as long as 20 or 30 months postpartum. This is perfectly normal and healthy. The three longest durations of amenorrhea recorded in our breastfeeding surveys were two at 42 months and one at 43 months. (They are not included in the 14.5 months' average.)

Of those doing ecological breastfeeding, about 93% will be in amenorrhea at 6 months postpartum, about 56% will be in amenorrhea at 12 months postpartum, and about 33% will still be in amenorrhea at 18 months postpartum. About 70% of ecological breastfeeding mothers will experience their first menstrual period between nine and 20 months postpartum.

Mothers who are well informed about natural family planning have found that even when their periods return early and they continued frequent and unrestricted nursing, they charted many infertile cycles. A few mothers who experience an early return of menstruation with ecological breastfeeding will not be fertile until their baby is about a year old. This is easily determined by charting and is common with mothers who keep up the ecological breastfeeding, lots of nursing and the family bed. Thus for these mothers under the natural mothering program, fertility is delayed considerably even though menstruation may be occurring regularly.

Those mothers who go for two years without any menstrual cycles due to nursing are not abnormal. Such extended lactation amenorrhea is common in certain cultures. One study among Eskimos showed that the mothers who nursed traditionally did not conceive until 20 to 30 months after childbirth, whereas the younger Eskimo mothers who adopted the American practices of supplements and bottlefeeding were conceiving within two to four months after childbirth.[3] When I wrote the first draft of this book, I felt that lactation amenorrhea of 12 months was exceptionally long. Of course, today that is on the short side of the average of 14.5 months. Since that time I have met many mothers who have experienced an absence of periods for 24 months after childbirth, so that this now sounds very normal. What is abnormal is having menstrual cycles return within three months after childbirth. Nature intended for women to have an extended period of amenorrhea so that babies would be spaced.

The return of fertility

Fertility generally returns around the time when menstruation resumes. That is why the return of menstruation is a good general indicator of the return of fertility. There are three exceptions: 1) a nursing mother does have a small chance of becoming fertile before her first menstruation; 2) as indicated already, some nursing mothers have a number of anovulatory cycles, especially if they have an early return of menstruation; and 3) a few nursing mothers may have regular "fertile" cycles according to her charts, but cannot become pregnant until all breastfeeding has ceased. This latter situation is why a mother should not seek fertility help while she is still nursing.

Demographic scientists know that ecological breastfeeding in the first six months of amenorrhea is one of the best methods of postponing pregnancy, but for some reason this information is silenced at the popular level. The American Academy of Pediatrics' "Policy Statement on Breastfeeding" listed eight proven benefits of breastfeeding for the woman. **Two** of the eight benefits dealt with breastfeeding infertility, but the contemporary press releases from three wire services plus local newspaper articles listing the women's benefits from this Statement failed to list these two benefits. For the record, the "Statement" says: "Lactational amenorrhea causes less menstrual blood loss over the months after delivery" and there is a "delayed resumption of ovulation with increased child spacing."[4]

What is the baby-spacing effectiveness of ecological breastfeeding while in amenorrhea? During the first three months of ecological breastfeeding and lactation amenorrhea, the probability of becoming pregnant is almost nil. During the next three months of amenorrhea and ecological breastfeeding, the chances of pregnancy are at the one percent level. The earliest return of fertility I've seen recorded by someone doing ecological breastfeeding was at 4½ months, based on her mucus and temperature record and followed by her first period. She always experienced an early return of fertility while breastfeeding, and she learned that her older relatives had the same experience. She took natural family planning classes and found the information to be very helpful. She had ample warning with the mucus and then had a good temperature shift. With abstinence according to the rules taught to this couple, they were able to postpone pregnancy and continue to nurse their baby.

After six months postpartum, the chance of becoming pregnant while doing ecological breastfeeding and still in amenorrhea is 6%. In these cases ovulation occurs prior to what would have been the first menstrual period if pregnancy had not occurred. That figure is based on several studies. In 1897, Remfry found a 5% pregnancy rate before the first period among Quebec breastfeeding mothers.[5] In 1969 Bonte and van Balem found a similar rate of 5.4% in Rwanda.[6] In 1971 Prem reported a rate of 6% among American breastfeeding mothers.[7]

For mothers who do not desire another pregnancy at this time and are concerned about the risk of pregnancy prior to the return of menstruation, proper instruction in natural family planning can reduce that risk to close to one percent.[8] For mothers desiring immediate pregnancy, I would still encourage natural family planning charting because the upward shift in temperatures right after ovulation is the best indicator of your baby's age during pregnancy. This evidence may save you unnecessary tests and expense; it may also prevent a premature induced delivery. Based on your chart your due date may be later than your doctor's due date which is based on the start of your last menstrual period or other indicators. Your "scientific" data would be more accurate. The temperature graph is the single most accurate method of estimating the date of conception and therefore gestational age, according to Dr. Konald Prem, professor emeritus of the Department of Obstetrics and Gynecology of the University of Minnesota School of Medicine...even more accurate than ultrasound.[9] The charting information is always helpful in estimating the date of childbirth, and it's even more important in high-risk pregnancies or complications. For the doctor who is concerned because he thinks you are overdue, the chart can either confirm his opinion or show otherwise.

The general experience of those mothers with long periods of lactation amenorrhea is that normal fertility is not impaired once menstruation returns or once the child is completely weaned. The mother who experienced 43 months of lactation amenorrhea was most appreciative of the information found in the first edition of this book: "I would have never suppressed ovulation for 3½ years," and "I could have wasted money and time in doctors' offices thinking I was abnormal." She found that once her cycles returned, they "have been quite regular and ovulation occurs each month." Many mothers also experience another pregnancy shortly after lactation amenorrhea ends, showing that fertility has not been impaired by the breastfeeding experience.

Two opposing but equally false statements about breastfeeding continue to obscure the truth. The first says, "Breastfeeding doesn't space babies." The second says, "You can't get pregnant while breastfeeding." This book and this chapter in particular aim to clarify the realities. First of all, only ***ecological*** breastfeeding normally provides any significant delay in the return of fertility. However, with the typical American *cultural* ways of restricted nursing, menstruation often returns about three months postpartum and fertility returns quickly as well. Second, even with ecological breastfeeding, most nursing mothers will have their fertility return while still nursing.

With proper knowledge and support, and with the practice of ecological breastfeeding, the average nursing mother will experience an extended period of infertility and a long absence from menstruation. If no form of conception regulation is used except ecological breastfeeding, babies will be spaced about two years apart, on the average.

[1] "Consensus Statement: Breastfeeding as a Family Planning Method," *Lancet*, November 19, 1988, 1204-5.

[2] See Chapter 21.

[3] J. Hildes and O. Schaefer, "Health of Igloolik Eskimos and Changes with Urbanization," Paper presented at the Circumpolar Health Symposium, Oulu, Finland, June 1971.

[4] American Academy of Pediatrics, "Policy Statement: Breastfeeding and the Use of Human Milk," *Pediatrics*, December 1997.

[5] L. Remfry, "The Effects of Lactation on Menstruation and Pregnation," *Transactions of the Obstetrical Society of London*, 38(1897), 22-27.

[6] M. Bonte and H. van Balem, "Prolonged Lactationand Family Spacing in Rwanda," *Journal of Biosocial Science*, April 1969, 97-100.

[7] Konald Prem, M.D., "Post-Partum Ovulation," Unpublished paper presented at the La Leche League International Conference, Chicago, July 1971.

[8] See Chapter 22.

[9] K. Prem, "Assessment of Gestational Age," *Minnesota Medicine*, Spetember 1976, 623.

Getting Off to a Good Start

The most successful breastfeeding and natural mothering experiences are those that get off to a good start. This is not to say that mothers who have gotten off to a poor start cannot have rewarding mothering experiences, but certainly it is more pleasant to have everything going for you from the beginning than to experience all sorts of problems.

There are various factors involved in getting off to a good start. Some have to do with the mental, educational, and physical preparation of the mother. Others have to do with the doctor or midwife, the childbirth experience, and advisors, whether freely chosen or self-appointed. Sometimes all of these favorably combine for a delightful experience. At other times a mother may have to be very determined and even courageous in order to have things working for her instead of against her.

The mother herself

In conversations about the desirability of breastfeeding and its naturalness, the first question that usually arises is, "What about the mother who can't nurse?" I think that those who are physically unable to breastfeed are about as rare as those who are physically unable to swim. A mother who has had both breasts surgically removed would obviously be physically unable to nurse her baby just as a person without arms or legs would be unable to swim. The vast majority of those mothers who can't nurse are in the same category as those who can't swim — they have never learned how. Also, if society looked down on the idea of girls swimming, we would have very few women swimmers. If society looks down on or at least does not encourage breastfeeding, we are going to have few women successfully breastfeeding.

For those few mothers who may not be able to nurse because of some unfortunate situation, much of the motherly advice in this book can still be followed. The philosophy of giving of yourself, being close and in touch with your child, taking him with you, holding him for the bottlefeedings, sleeping with him, enjoying and loving him are the best "gifts" you can give your small child. One mother looked upon bottlefeeding as a handicap.

I was mothering our first baby the "natural mothering" way but with a bottle because I thought I was unable to nurse. I experienced the identical sleep cycles. We napped together, slept together, and woke together continuously for the first year, although she did sleep at night in a crib when she turned 11 months. I told myself that bottlefeeding was like a handicap that I had to overcome. I would think that if *I* were a wheelchair-bound mother, I wouldn't be able to run with my child, but I could still have a rich, loving relationship. So, I looked upon my inability to breastfeed as a handicap to overcome. I am now breastfeeding our second baby and it is everything I had imagined. It has been sheer bliss.

There are many reasons given by mothers as to why they were unable to nurse. They had the desire, but they say: "I did not have enough milk," "My nipples were too sore," "My baby was not gaining weight," "My doctor told me to quit," "My doctor told me that I couldn't for medical reasons." The real reason why these mothers did not nurse is probably the lack of encouragement from someone who was familiar with this natural process and had the proper advice and information to share.

At La Leche League's (LLL) 1997 World Conference celebrating LLL's 40th anniversary, Dr. Jay Gordon spoke on "insufficient milk syndrome" which he said is a myth and which is really "insufficient advice." This California pediatrician says that if "insufficient milk syndrome" occurred in 1 out of 100 or even in 1 out of 1,000 mothers, he would see two or three cases a year and he doesn't. He claims mothers can nurse well with proper information and support, and he suggests a visit by a La Leche League leader or lactation consultant on the third day postpartum to make sure the breastfeeding is going well.[1]

Many nursing mothers are led to believe that their breastfed baby should be on a four-hour schedule. When baby cries two hours later, they begin to think their milk isn't good enough, or they worry and wonder why the baby isn't satisfied with a four-hour schedule. What these mothers don't realize is that their milk is well suited to the baby's digestive system, that breastmilk does not curd in the baby's stomach as formula milk does. Because breastmilk digests so much faster than formula milk, breastfeeding babies need to feed more often than every four hours.

Several couples have told me that they had to quit nursing because their baby had diarrhea. They have been misinformed. A doctor friend who is well read on the breastfed baby says that a baby does not have to be taken off the breast for any type of diarrhea unless the baby is so sick that he needs transfusions and couldn't nurse anyway. It is, in fact, the other way around. One mother whose baby had severe diarrhea was told by her doctor to exclusively breastfeed. Later, when the crisis was past, he told her she would have lost the baby if she had not been nursing.

Some mothers need to distinguish diarrhea from the soft liquid stool of a breastfed baby. This normal stool will remain a thick liquid up until the time the child begins solids. An exclusively breastfed baby was not meant to have a hard-formed stool. In addition, in the early days a baby may have several movements a day or a slight spotting with each feeding.

Later, couples begin to worry about the opposite; they fear the baby is constipated. As the baby gets older, he may at times have a bowel movement only once every two or three days. There may be a few times when he will go even seven days without a bowel movement, but the stool is very soft when it arrives. If a mother realizes that breastmilk is utilized very efficiently by the baby's body and that very little is eliminated as solid waste, she can understand why it might take several days for her baby to build up enough waste matter before there is adequate pressure for elimination.

There may also be a situation in which a doctor will tell the mother to quit nursing because of a drug or test that is required of the mother. It is extremely rare that a mother would have to quit nursing for medical reasons. Usually the nursing need only be stopped temporarily. Sometimes the procedure can wait until the baby is weaned.

Sometimes doctors are not well informed about a particular drug's effect upon a nursing baby, and they recommend weaning for safety purposes without seriously looking into the matter or without thinking of an alternative solution. For example, a close friend who was hospitalized and taking three medications was told by her doctor to wean her older baby from the breast. She was very upset with this advice. I encouraged her to call a local doctor who happened to be on the La Leche League Medical Advisory Board. Acting on my advice, she learned that she could continue to take all three medications and continue the breastfeeding as well.

Sometimes we are at fault because we fail to seek a second opinion. The mother who encouraged me to write this book weaned because she was scheduled to have a radioactive thyroid test; the doctors insisted on complete weaning before the test. Both she and her toddler were miserable during the two-week weaning period. She became painfully engorged; her little one was upset and frequently in tears. This mother had always been very active in her local La Leche League group, often acting as librarian. Through her local group, she later found out that weaning was not necessary, that the nursing only had to be stopped for a short time. Why hadn't she thought to contact La Leche League right away? It never occurred to her! Oftentimes we assume the experts are knowledgeable, and we never think to question their decisions. When she learned she had weaned unnecessarily, this mother was even more upset because she had failed to look into the matter and regretted the complete and abrupt weaning decision.

Besides contacting La Leche League to determine whether breastfeeding can be continued or not, you might find your answer in Dr. Thomas Hale's book, *Medications and Mothers' Milk*.[2] He updates his book yearly and his expertise has been nationally recognized. One of our daughters found his book very helpful when considering medications after surgery; she was concerned about the possible effects upon her nursing baby. Therefore, if any problem does develop for you or your nursing baby, you are now better informed as to your choices. And it may be as easy as looking up your specific situation in the LLL manual, *The Womanly Art of Breastfeeding*.[3]

Nursing may be hard to establish if the mother has lots of company. A new mother should not have to spend time entertaining people. Any relative who stays with your family after childbirth should be pro-breastfeeding. I have one friend who could not get the breastfeeding established in the presence of her visiting mother. With her third baby, she decided to invite her mother only *after* the breastfeeding was already going well. With that baby, she was very happy to exclusively breastfeed and later considered it a pleasure to wonder when her baby would start solids.

Many parents are supportive, and for that we are most thankful. However, a common complaint among many nursing mothers is that their mother or mother-in-law is opposed to their nursing or especially opposed to the nursing as the baby grows older. In these situations, it is important for the mother to have the support of her husband and other nursing-mother friends. Her husband can also handle the responses for his wife. Sometimes joking is the only solution: "We know he'll start solids by kindergarten," or "I'm sure he will wean before high school." Your husband's support is invaluable, especially when the negative remarks and questioning are coming from his family.

A mother who desires to breastfeed should be well informed so that she is likely to have a successful nursing experience. Her learning process should start during the months before childbirth by attending the meetings of the La Leche League or other associations of nursing mothers. The mother-to-be should read the La Leche League manual, *The Womanly Art of Breastfeeding*.

La Leche League has a professional board of medical advisors plus the experience of thousands of women. Many mothers are most appreciative for the help and information they have received from this organization. Having the right answer and support at the right time can mean success instead of failure.

Young mothers today may also lack confidence in themselves. These mothers only require a little more time to develop the self-confidence they need. It does take a little while for a first-time mother to forget about rules and time schedules, and until this happens the mother does not really relax and enjoy nursing her baby. At any rate, all that most of these mothers need is a lot of praise and someone telling them that they are doing what is best for their baby.

Another benefit of sleeping with your baby during the night and for a nap is that many breastfeeding problems may be avoided as the baby nurses for a long time on one or both breasts. Rest and good drainage of the breast by the baby during these sleep times can eliminate severe plugged ducts. Some mothers experience hard substances called "milk crystals" near the nipple surface that plug the milk flow of a particular duct and these have to be expelled. A doctor friend has had these substances with each baby and claims that the situation is helped only by sleeping with her baby at least once during the day or during the night.

The doctor

What is the role of the physician in breastfeeding? Certainly, his influence is considerable with most mothers. He is therefore in an excellent position to foster the practice of breastfeeding and natural mothering. He can explain to the mother how her milk is the best food for the baby. He can tell her all the health advantages to both the baby and herself through breastfeeding. He can tell her about natural mothering and the natural infertility of ecological breastfeeding. He can assure her that she will be able to do a good job. He can recommend she attend the La Leche League meetings during pregnancy. He can give parents a copy of the "Policy Statement on Breastfeeding" by the American Academy of Pediatrics.

If you already have a relationship of long standing with a particular doctor, you may want to stay with him even if he's not as informed and supportive as you might wish. If he knows you, he may be quite interested in your new ideas. One mother expressed concern about her doctor's reaction to exclusive breastfeeding since he had put her previous babies on solids within several weeks after birth. She later told me that he went along with her although he mentioned solids at each visit, but he jokingly told her, "You know more about it than I." Understandably, that same doctor may be less open to new ideas from a total stranger. Other mothers may present the AAP "Policy Statement on Breastfeeding" to their doctors since this Statement provides the research to show what is best for the breastfed baby.

The childbirth experience

Under healthy, normal, natural conditions, a new baby should be nursing within a few minutes after childbirth and before the cord is cut. This is just as much for the mother's benefit as for his own because the baby's suckling helps her uterus to contract and to close the maternal blood vessels that formerly took care of him. In brief, that means that your baby's suckling helps to prevent hemorrhaging, and your baby receives more iron as the cord continues to pulsate blood toward the baby. Your baby's continued suckling in the next 24 to 48 hours gives him the benefits of a fluid called colostrum, the first milk secreted by the breast. It is much richer and creamier than the milk that soon follows.

I cannot emphasize too strongly that a mother should allow her baby to breastfeed without restriction during the first 24 hours after childbirth. If you want a successful nursing experience, start early. Don't be surprised if your baby doesn't nurse a minute or so after his birth. He will do better a few minutes later. At a *minimum*, your baby should be allowed to nurse within the first half-hour after birth. Preferably the baby will be allowed to remain in bed with you, and he can nurse on and off to his heart's content. More hospitals are keeping the baby with mother from the time of the baby's birth, and more hospitals are adopting policies that are more conducive to successful nursing — no artificial nipples for breastfeeding babies.

In order for mother and baby to have this good start at nursing, they both should be physically able right after the birth. Thus I recommend a prepared and, if possible, a completely unmedicated childbirth as the best for a successful breastfeeding experience. A baby may be adversely affected by any drug used on the mother and may not be inclined toward nursing. Hopefully the mother can begin nursing right after birth with an alert, undrugged baby. That in turn means she has to have a physician who will, first of all, allow her to nurse after childbirth.

The next thing she normally needs from her physician is the *absence* of a shot to contract her uterus; baby's suckling takes care of that. Unfortunately, some mothers have to shop around before they can find a doctor who is agreeable and who will not intervene in the natural process unless truly needed.

Another option is to hire a doula for support during labor at the hospital, especially in areas where medicated births are extremely high. One of our daughters was so grateful for the services of her doula that she and her husband sent the doula a bouquet of flowers in appreciation. Some mothers seek the services of a midwife for birthing at home, at the hospital, or at a birthing center. Many obstetricians and more hospitals now offer midwife services in a given practice or health-care plan.

Your doctor's Cesarean section rate

An expectant couple would do well to ask any doctor who might be present at the birth of their child what his C-section rate is. According to the Public Citizen Health Research Group which is affiliated with the Ralph Nader organization, 455,000 C-sections were done unnecessarily in 1986. They also claim that "the national C-section rate has more than quadrupled in the last 16 years."[4] Most of the variations in the C-section rate, the group found, were due to the various policies of physicians and hospitals. For example, I know of one local physician who told a laboring mother as she entered the hospital, "If you don't have the baby in ten hours, we'll do a C-section." A doctor who did a C-section on a close friend of mine told her prior to the surgery that he had to get back to his patients. Consumers (those having babies) should become better informed so they will be in a better position to protect themselves. Hospitals and doctors should provide their C-section rate to any consumer upon request. In the fall of 1998, I was surprised to see a billboard in eastern Ohio advertising a local hospital's low C-section rate!

Vertical birthing

An upright or vertical position during labor and birthing certainly facilitates labor and birthing, and I think it can also reduce the C-section rate. Connie Livingston points out that "a position such as squatting can ease the process by increasing the opening of your pelvic bones as much as .5 to 2.5 centimeters."[5] Other benefits include less tearing, improved fetal blood supply and less need for intervention. Regarding less tearing and episiotomies, those who have had both an episiotomy and then experienced a slight tear without the episiotomy usually find that it is easier on the body and less painful to experience a slight tear with its appropriate repair than to undergo another episiotomy. The vertical position is more comfortable and easier for the mother-to-be as she has gravity working for her. With labor usually shortened, she has more energy as well.

By upright position, I do not mean the flat-on-your back position with your head or shoulders slightly elevated. I mean that your body torso is in a vertical position for labor and birthing. Vertical positions include sitting, standing, kneeling, and squatting.

One of the best and very attractive brochures that I have seen on this topic is "Squatting: The Position for Labor and Birth" by Megan Steelman. It lists 24 benefits of squatting and, in fairness, lists three disadvantages or cautions for squatting. The squatting positions fall into two categories: the full squat or the standing squat. A total of eleven positions are described and illustrated.[6]

Other advisors

In addition to medical doctors, a mother may seek and receive advice about breastfeeding, parenting, or family planning from other persons, such as her clergyman, her mother-in-law, or a teacher. Schools, colleges, and churches may offer courses on marriage and family life, and frequently they have the opportunity to touch upon these topics. At the least, these sources should not discourage the natural plan for mother and baby and natural child spacing. More affirmatively, they should know enough about ecological breastfeeding to be able to describe what is involved, and they can encourage couples to attend the natural family planning classes taught by the Couple to Couple League. These classes may be the only place where couples will gain the proper information about ecological breastfeeding and systematic natural family planning through fertility awareness. Couples who cannot attend the classes can learn natural family planning in the privacy of their home through the *CCL Home Study Course.*[7] Teachers and the clergy can have a great influence upon the young and upon couples preparing for marriage. Many couples will appreciate their guidance in this area of their lives.

Various marriage and family courses and conferences provide an excellent opportunity to educate people who are open and receptive to the ideas of natural breastfeeding — men as well as women. Yes, men need to learn all the advantages of breastfeeding since the understanding and encouragement of a husband is invaluable to the nursing mother.

In our society, if the case for breastfeeding and natural mothering were made with the same emphasis given to the bottle, baby foods, the pill and other unnatural forms of birth control, I feel that the desires of many mothers to breastfeed would remain alive. Many couples do not consider breastfeeding because they are never presented with any reasons for doing so. A renewed effort by all the related professions to impart factual information about this natural process could change that picture.

Support

Where does a couple find support and information with regard to breastfeeding and the natural spacing of babies? Couples who are interested in getting off to a good start can find support and information from two nonprofit organizations, each of which has its own specialty. Each is listed in the "Resources" section at the end of this book.

The Couple to Couple League International (CCL)

Natural family planning (NFP) is the specialty of CCL. CCL classes are available throughout the United States and in over 20 foreign countries. Since breastfeeding is the world's oldest form of natural family planning, CCL has long been interested in promoting ecological breastfeeding. The natural family planning classes are taught by professionally trained volunteer user-couples; a home study course is available for those who cannot attend classes. The learner's manual, *The Art of Natural Family Planning*, is available in English, Czech, Dutch, French, Hungarian, Polish, Russian, and Spanish. In the classes and in *The Art of Natural Family Planning*, couples will learn about ecological breastfeeding and about systematic natural family planning. The bi-monthly CCL magazine, *CCL Family Foundations*, receives high praise from many couples.

La Leche League International (LLL)

This organization is dedicated to helping mothers learn "the womanly art of breastfeeding": hence, the title of its manual. La Leche League chapters are located in many towns and cities throughout the United States and other countries. The ideal time for a woman to complete the regular series of meetings given by the League is during pregnancy. The League's manual, *The Womanly Art of Breastfeeding*, is a book every nursing mother should have in her possession to read and reread as needed.

A Review of my recommendations

1. Read *The Art of Natural Family Planning*. Attend the Couple to Couple League (CCL) classes on natural family planning or take the *CCL Home Study Course*.

2. Read *The Womanly Art of Breastfeeding*.

3. Read childbirth books and take local childbirth classes taught by a midwife, doula, or childbirth educator.

4. Choose your doctors carefully. Write down your important questions and bring your list with you. Have your husband come with you if you feel the need for support.

5. Remember you have a right to have the natural care that is best for you and your baby, and you can feel secure knowing that "science" is there for the unusual circumstance should you or the baby require special treatment.

6. Since "natural" in man does not mean the same as "automatic," you have a corresponding duty to prepare yourself ahead of time both intellectually and physically in order to fully assist the natural processes. Don't expect a natural-type childbirth experience without adequate childbirth preparation and planning. Don't expect a successful nursing experience without learning something about breastfeeding. Attend meetings offered by La Leche League if possible.

7. Learn with your husband whenever possible. Share with him anything new that you've learned about breastfeeding and other related issues. Attend childbirth classes, breastfeeding or family conferences, and natural family planning classes together. Babies are always welcome at the Couple to Couple League classes or events, and I know the same goes for the La Leche League meetings and conferences.

To conclude, I would like to add that many of us who have breastfed owe a deep debt of gratitude to a particular doctor or nurse who gave us the proper support and advice about childbirth and breastfeeding. If your doctor or hospital is less than ideal, you need to realize that most hospitals and doctors practice as they do because that is what their patients want. Some mothers want to start their babies on solids early or want to use the bottle. Some mothers want to be fully medicated during the birth process. Some mothers or parents look to science to solve all their problems. There are some doctors who would like to see a change, but they are faced with the difficult job of reeducating their patients as to what is best for them. Some doctors will personally recommend breastfeeding or natural childbirth only to have a woman respond negatively. She just isn't interested.

Both the childbirth and early breastfeeding experiences are interrelated and play an important part in the mother-baby ecology. If this ecology is disturbed during childbirth and the immediate postpartum hours, then the breastfeeding may not get off to a good start. I hope you can take the steps recommended in this chapter so that your breastfeeding experience gets off to the best start possible.

[1] Jay Gordon, "Insufficient Milk Syndrome," LLLI World Conference, July 1997; 410-643-4220.

[2] T. Hale, *Medications and Mothers' Milk.* Available through CCL, 800-745-8252 (orders only).

[3] LLLI, *The Womanly Art of Breastfeeding.* Available through CCL.

[4] "450,000 C-Sections Called Unnecessary," *The Cincinnati Post*, November 2, 1987.

[5] C. Livingston, "Birth in the Squatting Position," *Maternal Health News*, December 2, 1988, 2.

[6] M. Steelman, "Squatting," *Childbirth Graphics.* Available through CCL.

[7] CCL, *Home Study Course.* Available through CCL.

The First Six Months

Few parents are aware of *all* the specific advantages of breastfeeding exclusively during the first six months of a baby's life. This chapter encourages and reinforces you in your desire to nurse your baby and to offer him nothing but your milk during at least the first six months of life.

Nature's product: the best

Your milk is the best food you can give your baby. Breastmilk has all the calories, proteins, vitamins, water, and other essential elements needed for your baby's growth — except Vitamin D which a baby's body makes from exposure to sunlight. Nature, which did a fantastic job of nurturing and developing new life within your body for nine months before birth, has likewise provided a completely nutritious food for your baby's growth after birth. Nature intends a continuity between the nourishment you gave your baby in your womb and the nourishment you can give your baby at your breasts. In fact, so great is this continuity that even if you should have a preterm baby, your milk is adjusted accordingly.

From the baby's point of view, unrestricted nursing from the very beginning may be quite important for his health. The secretion that comes from a mother's breast at birth, the colostrum, is different from and richer than the milk that will soon follow. This first milk is valuable to an infant's health, for cells present in colostrum ingest and destroy bacteria. This infection-fighting quality continues with the day-to-day and month-to-month and even year-to year production of breastmilk. Colostrum changes to meet the changing needs of your baby. The colostrum of the first day is not the same as the colostrum of the second day, and no formula can duplicate these changes day by day or even hour by hour. When the transitional milk starts coming in, there are similar changes to meet the needs of the baby, and breastmilk continues to change as the baby ages. Breastmilk is indeed a **living** food.

Of course, you need to provide yourself with good nutrition. The maternal diet is important in order for your baby to derive the greatest benefit from the ecological relationship. Therefore, during the months of pregnancy and during the months of breastfeeding, you should take special care to select proper foods for yourself and your family.

91

At birth the full-term baby has his own supply of iron which normally lasts until the time of gradual introduction of other foods. If you exclusively breastfeed for six months and continue breastfeeding for at least one year, your baby will not need iron supplementation, according to Dr. Alfredo Pisacane, an Italian pediatrician and researcher. What about the breastfed baby who does not want solids after six months of age? Dr. Pisacane has found no anemia in babies breastfed exclusively for eight or nine months and sees no reason to test a breastfed baby for iron at 12 months if he is taking enough solid food. This doctor claims that "prolonged breastfeeding and a delayed cord clamping" are a cheap and effective solution for the prevention of iron-deficiency anemia." He also questions the levels of iron used to measure anemia: "Who says 12.5 grams of iron is better than 11 grams or who says 11 grams of iron is better than 10.6 grams? Nobody knows." Then he hinted that nature knows best since too much iron in the baby's bowel can increase the growth of bacteria. As an example, he said that if you treat malaria in Africa with iron, the malaria gets worse.[1]

Other researchers have reported "that a great majority of exclusively breastfed infants are able to maintain their iron status at the same level as that of control infants receiving iron supplements"; they "could not demonstrate any anemia in infants after exclusive breastfeeding for nine months." They concluded that their data "indicate that it is safe, in exclusively breastfed infants, to shift the starting age for iron supplementation to six months, or even older."[2]

Exclusively breastfed babies can appear obese as babies and this may concern parents. However, a physician friend of ours who promotes breastfeeding has seen many obese babies — breastfed and bottlefed. He claims that there is a big difference between obesity due to bottlefeeding and that due to breastfeeding. As they become active, walking and running toddlers, the bottlefed youngster tends to retain his heaviness while the breastfed youngster slims down in appearance.

Many of us who promote breastfeeding have been acquainted with babies who require special formulas, which can be quite costly. This expense, of course, might have been avoided if the mother had been exclusively breastfeeding in the first place. There are also a few babies who would have died if breastmilk had not been available to them. I would like to quote from two letters I received while in the process of writing this book.

> Our league here has just had a rewarding experience in providing breastmilk for a very premature baby who could not tolerate formula and [his condition] was becoming very critical. The pediatrician called La Leche League as a last resort since the mother was not nursing. After being given breastmilk, the baby improved immediately and surpassed his birth weight of slightly over two pounds.

Right now we are supplying a baby with breastmilk. He was three and a half months old and barely living at eight pounds in the University Hospital at Saskatoon when I was asked if we could provide breastmilk for him. Now (a month later) he is a healthy 11 pounds 14 ounces and growing at an unbelievable rate. The mother is trying to relactate but is having quite a bit of difficulty. There is no doubt that this baby would have died had he not gotten breastmilk.

Doctors N. W. Wilson and R. N. Hamburger noted that between 2% and 3% of the general population of infants are allergic to cow's milk but that such allergy may reach the 30 percent level among children who inherit allergic tendencies from their parents. The treatment is common sense: "Avoidance [of cow's milk] is the mainstay of treatment and breastfeeding is the optimal choice," and that means "exclusive breastfeeding for about six months combined with delayed introduction to solid foods for at least six months."[3] This makes good sense for all, for who can foresee what child will inherit allergic tendencies?

Exclusive breastfeeding saves "work" time, time that isn't spent in the kitchen preparing bottles, nipples, and formula or spent cleaning up afterwards. Breastfeeding does take time, but it's more in the form of nurturing, time better spent with the baby.

Breastmilk is always ready and available and at the right temperature. Breastfeeding means "little breaks" during the day to sit down (or lie down) and enjoy the baby God gave you. It's less work for the sick mother who can care for her baby in bed. It is probably less work for the physically handicapped mother who would also enjoy this intimate contact with her baby. It means having one arm and hand free to hug another child, answer the phone, or eat a meal. Breastfeeding generally means fewer visits to the doctor or hospital. It also means easier travel, whether it's a day outing for

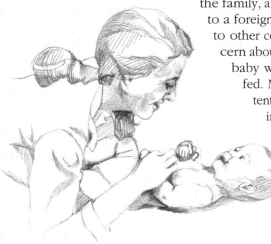

the family, a week's vacation, or a trip to a foreign country. When traveling to other countries, there is no concern about foods and water for the baby who is exclusively breastfed. My husband and I, being tent campers, found that tenting and hiking was easy with a breastfed baby.

Breastfeeding saves money. Obviously, one does not have to buy bottles, nipples, brushes, sterilizer, formula, pacifiers, juice, and baby food. Money is also

93

saved by not having to buy sanitary supplies during the months of lactation amenorrhea. Breastfeeding means less money spent on doctors' fees, hospital expenses, and probably fewer drugs and fewer dental bills because statistically your child will be healthier.

Couples who use ecological breastfeeding and systematic natural family planning (NFP) will also save time and money by eliminating visits to the doctor for prescription birth control plus its regular checkup visits, special visits due to side effects, and for a switch to another method, or possible future surgery. The amount of money involved is indicated by a doctor's statement that he forfeited $30,000 a month in his practice of obstetrics/gynecology when he became an NFP-only physician.[4]

Nursing mothers have calculated that when a mother exclusively breastfeeds for the first six months postpartum, the money saved will easily buy a basic king-size bed. A headboard is not necessary; we have never used one. I suggest you use those savings to purchase such a bed. It makes sleeping with your baby much, much easier.

Does nature have a diet plan for your baby? I think so. The presence of a strong sucking reflex and the absence of teeth are physical signs indicating that nature intended babies to have milk in the first months of life. When I was training to be a dental hygienist, we were taught that the first set of teeth were called milk teeth in the past. That did not make sense to me as a college student having had no exposure to breastfeeding. However, considering the natural plan for prolonged lactation, I easily see now why they were called milk teeth. These teeth begin to come in around the middle of the baby's first year. At about this time the baby's hand coordination is better and he is beginning to put things in his mouth. Soon he will be ready for a gradual introduction of solid food while he continues to take only breastmilk for his liquid diet. Giving the baby under six months of age early foods or liquids means that the baby is getting less and less of good breastmilk. Again, normally the baby under six months needs only breastmilk. Nothing else is needed.

The emotional benefits of breastfeeding should be valued as much as the physical benefits of breastfeeding. More and more emphasis is being placed on the importance of skin-to-skin contact between parent and child — whether it be in the act of nursing a baby, rubbing a child's back, or rocking a child to sleep. Physical contact generates warm feelings of being loved and appreciated. Exclusive breastfeeding guarantees that the child will receive frequent contact with his mother during the first six months of life. Nature continues to ensure this physical and emotional nurturing through prolonged lactation.

What happens to a mother during those first six months? First, she is discovering that breastfeeding is generally a very satisfying and enjoyable experience for her. She is also learning how to be a good mother in an easy environment. Through breastfeeding she learns to sacrifice her desires and time for her child's benefit. Oh yes, there will be difficult times when she has to nurse and comfort her baby for long periods of time. Yet she accepts this inconvenience because in her heart she knows that it is the right thing to do.

Medically recognized benefits

In December 1997 the American Academy of Pediatrics (AAP) issued a strong policy statement on "Breastfeeding and the Use of Human Milk" in which the Academy recommended that the new mother nurse exclusively for the first six months and that breastfeeding "continue for at least 12 months, and thereafter for as long as mutually desired." The AAP claimed "human milk is uniquely superior for infant feeding" even in "***developed*** countries" and reported a number of proven benefits and possible protective benefits of breastfeeding. In support of its policy, the statement listed over 100 scientific studies.[5]

The definitely ***proven*** benefits to the baby, according to the AAP, are that breastfeeding "***decreases the incidence and/or severity of***

- diarrhea
- lower respiratory infection
- otitis media [inner ear infection]
- bacteremia [bacteria in the blood stream]
- bacterial meningitis
- botulism
- urinary tract infection and
- necrotizing enterocolitis [part of the bowel dies and has to be sectioned out]."

The Statement also listed eight benefits for the baby that have not yet been thoroughly proven. These are called ***possible*** protective effects from breastfeeding. There is a possibility that breastfeeding offers protection from the following:

- sudden infant death syndrome
- insulin-dependent diabetes mellitus
- Crohn's disease
- ulcerative colitis
- lymphoma
- allergic diseases and
- other chronic digestive diseases.
- Breastfeeding may also enhance "cognitive development."

The AAP lists eight benefits for the mother who breastfeeds:

- less postpartum bleeding
- more rapid uterine involution
- less menstrual blood loss over the months after delivery [very familiar to readers of this book]
- an earlier return to prepregnant weight
- delayed resumption of ovulation with increased child spacing

[also familiar to readers of this book]
- improved bone remineralization postpartum with reduction in hip fractures in the postmenopausal period
- reduced risk of ovarian cancer
- reduced risk of premenopausal breast cancer.

The goal of the American Academy of Pediatrics is to have 50% of new mothers in America breastfeeding at six months postpartum by the year 2000. When this report was issued, only 20% of American new mothers were still nursing at six months postpartum, and many of these mothers were using supplementation or formula. This Policy Statement makes it clear that the AAP wants most mothers to offer only breastmilk to their babies under six months of age.

---

[1] Alfredo Piscane, "Reconsidering the Timing of Solids," LLLI World Conference, July 1997; 410-643-4220.

[2] M. Simes et al., "Exclusive Breastfeeding For Nine Months: Risk of Iron Deficiency," *Pediatrics*, 104:2 (1984), 199.

[3] N. Wilson and R. Hamburger, "Allergy to Cow's Milk in the First Year of Life and Its Prevention," *Annals of Allergy*, November 1988, 323-27.

[4] Paul Hayes interviewed by Radix, "Birth Control," audiotape, Summer 1997.

[5] AAP, "Breastfeeding and Human Milk," *Pediatrics*, December 1997, 1035-39.

12

The Crucial First Three Years

A young mother finishing her college education was wondering if she really had to stay home when she had children. Wouldn't she be wasting the money she spent on her education and career? Wouldn't she be bored staying at home? She was asking for my advice. The day after I received her letter I met an old friend at a homeschooling event. This friend had worked full-time as a pharmacist with her first baby. Then over the years she had two more babies and went from a full-time pharmacist to part-time and eventually remained home. I told her about the letter and asked for her advice. Immediately she said, "Sheila, she has to find out for herself. Nothing you say will help." Maybe she was right, but I did try to encourage the inquiring mother to stay home once she had children. And I'm hopeful that this chapter might help more mothers and fathers to understand better the importance of the mother in the home. I include fathers because many husbands enjoy the wife's income, and a husband can be a decisive factor as to whether his wife stays home with their children or not.

Some expert opinion

My research over the years leads me to believe that what I'm calling natural mothering or ecological breastfeeding is at the heart of providing the best experience for the baby during the first three years of life. Why? Ecological breastfeeding keeps the mother with her baby during those important early years, and the mother learns to care for her baby using the equipment God gave her. The importance of that good start in life is emphasized by Dr. Burton White, director of the Parent Education Center in Newton, Massachusetts, who has spent over 40 years researching what causes competent people to get that way:

> On the basis of years of research, I am totally convinced that the first priority with respect to helping each child to reach his maximum level of competence is to do the best possible job in structuring his experience and opportunities during the first three years of life.[1]

Dr. John Bowlby, in his book on maternal deprivation, *Child Care and the Growth of Love*,[2] states that parents should not leave any child under three for several days unless for grave reason. If the mother must leave, someone close to the child should be chosen to care for the child.

Maria Montessori, who dedicated her later life to the study and education of young children, was one hundred percent in favor of natural mothering. In her fascinating and widely-read book, *The Absorbent Mind,* she encouraged only breastmilk for the first six months and told mothers to take their time with weaning. In fact, she recommended nursing for a year and a half to three years because "prolonged lactation requires the mother to remain with her child," and she promoted the practice of mother-baby inseparability during the early years.

> But let us think, for a moment, of the many peoples of the world who live at different cultural levels from our own. In the matter of child rearing, almost all of these seem to be more enlightened than ourselves — with all our Western ultramodern ideals... Mother and child are one. Except where civilization has broken down this custom, no mother ever entrusts her child to someone else.[3]

Selma Fraiberg, professor of Child Psychoanalysis at the University of Michigan Medical Center, also credits lactation as part of nature's way to keep mother and baby together.

> The breast was "intended" to bind the baby and his mother for the first year or two of life. If we read the biological program correctly, the period of breastfeeding insured continuity of mothering as part of the program for the formation of human bonds... A baby who is stored like a package with neighbors and relatives while his mother works may come to know as many indifferent caretakers as a baby in the lowest-grade institution and, at the age of one or two years, can resemble in all significant ways the emotionally deprived babies of such an institution.[4]

To stress the importance of the mother's presence during the early years, some authors and experts have made extremely impressive statements to show the effects of separation upon the child. Here are a few samples:

> If we assume that the sixth leading cause of death in the United States and the third leading cause of death in adolescence is not an inherited affliction, suicide must have its beginning in early life experiences. In the first eight months of life, an infant puts all its eggs into one basket, in the basket of the mother or surrogate mother, that I call "thee one," the one no one else will do for that infant... It's my contention that the first introduction to wish to be dead is when mother is not there and is not available.[5]

Edgar Draper, M.D.
Chairman of Psychiatry Department
University of Mississippi Medical Center

Full-time daycare, particularly group care, is especially harmful for children under the age of three. For two years we watched daycare children in our preschool/daycare center respond to the stresses of eight to ten hours a day of separation from their parents with tears, anger, withdrawal, or profound sadness, and we found, to our dismay, that nothing in our own affection and caring for these children would erase this sense of loss and abandonment. We came to realize that the amount of separation — the number of hours a day spent away from the parents — is a critical factor.[6]

William and Wendy Dreskin
Former daycare providers

The child's social development is always retarded if the child does not have a single main mother figure constantly about him, i.e., a person who has enough time and motherly love for the child. In this sentence, every word is equally important. **Single** does not mean two, three or four persons. **Constant** means always the same person. **Motherly** means a person who shows all of the behavior toward the child which we designate as "motherly." **Main mother figure** means that secondary mother figures (father, brothers, sisters, grandparents) may support the main mother figure, but may not substitute for her. **Person** means that the respective adult has to support the child with his whole being and has to have time for the child (emphasis in original).[7]

Theodore Hellbrügge
Director of Kindercentrum
Munich, Germany

There are six reactions of children to separation when the mother is not around her child. The pattern may be 1) depression, 2) agitation or distress, 3) rejection, 4) apathy, 5) regression or 6) clinging. Why would a mother do that to her child?... When can a child withstand separation from the mother? Up to two years of age is a high anxiety time; from two to three years of age is a lesser anxiety time. This varies with the individual.[8]

Hugh Riordan
Specialist in Human Communications
Director, The Olive W. Garvey Center of Human Functioning
Wichita, Kansas

There is no question from all the research that the risk of exploitation for a child increases directly as the child is removed further from the care of its biological mother. There is a population of child predators who will grab any opportunity to gain access to a child.[9]

Ronald Summit, M.D.
UCLA Psychiatrist

These experts are trying to show the possible effects upon the child when his mother is not there for him. It must also be noted that a stay-at-home mother can be extremely busy with other activities and ignore her baby's or other children's needs and responses. Maybe she is extremely preoccupied with cooking, cleaning house, doing volunteer work, conversing on the phone, watching television, or spending time on the Internet. It is one thing to take a few brief phone calls during the day; it is another to spend hours on the phone or at the computer at the expense of little ones. I'm not criticizing the mother who has the occasional long phone call and nurses her baby in the process. I'm only pointing out that any excessive activity at home that does not involve the children may mean neglecting one's duties as a mother. As one author appropriately said, "Busyness cancels out 'all-hereness'." In her book, *Your Child's Self-Esteem*, Dorothy Corkville Briggs further explains:

> The opposite of love is not hate, as many believe, but rather **indifference**. Nothing communicates disinterest more clearly than distancing. A child cannot feel valued by parents who are forever absorbed in their own affairs. Remember: distancing makes children feel unloved. No matter how we slice it, doses of genuine encounter pound home a vital message. Direct, personal involvement says, "It's important to me to be **with you**." On the receiving end, the child concludes, "I **must** matter because my folks take time to be involved with **my person**" (emphasis in original).[10]

Kathleen Parker warned working parents not to "delude themselves into thinking their day-care kids are doing fine simply because they 'seem' to be. Children don't necessarily give outward signs of distress at early ages. They don't suddenly start stammering or crying for no reason (though some do) or maiming small animals. The effects of low parental interest show up later — on the shrink's couch or the police blotter." She questions why we ignore the obvious, that kids need quantity time with their parents and ample nurturing during the first three years of life. Instead of a parent being home to nurture his child, the parent leaves home to find "solace and nurturing in the workplace."[11]

A psychotherapist compares the effects upon a small child when a total stranger takes care of him to the lack of care of one spouse for another spouse. Isabelle Fox says, "How important would any married person feel if his or her spouse was seldom home when needed or paid a stranger to take him or her out for dinner [or] to a movie?" The child taken care of by others similarly feels he is of little value to his parents. Dr. Fox asks, "Is there a noticeable difference in the child parented by a consistent, nurturing caregiver in the crucial pre-verbal years (0-3 years of age)?" She answers "Yes! During my 35 years as a psychotherapist, I have seen the benefits of a consistent, responsive caregiver and the disasters when this does not occur."[12]

Brain studies

In the spring of 1997 new studies showed that "the neurological foundation for problem solving and reasoning are largely established by age 1" and that the "number of words an infant hears each day from an attentive, engaged person is the single most important predictor of later intelligence, school success and social competence."[13] The studies emphasized that the number of words a baby hears during the first year of life must come from an "attentive, engaged human being." Discussion centered on the importance of the parents' role in the intellectual development of their child during the first three years of life and especially the first year of life when the infant's brain is growing at a tremendous rate.

As a result of the above studies, there was a renewed interest in Ohio about raising public awareness of the importance of the first three years of life. Dr. Gary Weisenberger, representing the Ohio Chapter of the American Academy of Pediatrics, encouraged parents to "play with their young children, read and sing to them, and spend more quality interactive time" because "now, new scientific evidence focuses on the importance of the first three years of a child's life" for his reading skills. And, he added, pediatricians know these early years are crucial to "other developmental and emotional factors that have a far-reaching effect on the child."[14]

Do language skills learned during the early years determine whether we develop Alzheimer's disease? In November of 1997, at the annual Rhode Island chapter of the Alzheimer's Association, Dr. David Snowdon reported on a study of 678 nuns. Of particular interest was one nun who died at age 87, mentally sharp until her death. When they looked at her brain, it was "riddled with tangles and plaques characteristic of Alzheimer's disease." (Those who had clumping and snarling of the brain nerve cells were more likely to have Alzheimer's if they had a stroke. Those less likely to develop Alzheimer's were those nuns who had Alzheimer's lesions but no strokes or those nuns with strokes but no Alzheimer's lesions.)

The nuns all wrote autobiographies at the time they entered the convent, and these written accounts were studied by the researchers. Of interest to them was the fact that those nuns who wrote with few ideas and in simple sentences were more likely to develop Alzheimer's. According to Dr. Snowdon, "It's more likely that the nuns' linguistic ability indicated how well their minds had developed early in life — and that optimal brain development in childhood can protect against Alzheimer's in old age."[15] If this is true, then nurturing that influences the growth of the brain for babies and children could also affect the brain's functioning as it ages.

Earlier I referred to studies that have linked language development to the type of care the child under three received from his parents. Dr. Burton White stressed the importance of the first three years of life for the emotional, intellectual, and linguistic development of the child. Development in all three areas depends upon the parent being willing to invest the necessary time. In his own words with respect to the development of language, Dr. White said: "It has been known for years that by three years of age, the average child will understand two-thirds to three-fourths of all the language he'll use for the rest of his life. It is also well known that language depends on experience."[16] And what is the best experience for the baby? According to Dr. White, it's the concentrated interaction with one parent during the first three years of life. Such experts and studies keep telling parents that their children will have better brain growth and language development if they, the parents, give hours of nurturing during the crucial first three years.

Other brain research has focused on the effects that breastmilk or breast-feeding has on a child's intelligence. For example, preemies who were fed breastmilk by tube had a 8.3 point advantage in IQ (Intelligence Quotient) at age 7½ to 8 years of age over those children of the same age who as preemies were fed no maternal milk by tube.[17] Two groups of phenylketo-nuric children were studied: those who had been exclusively breastfed and those fed formula. After adjusting for the differences in social category and maternal education, there was an overall advantage of 12.9 IQ points for the breastfed group.[18]

Does breastfeeding have any effect upon the child's academics during the grade school years and the high school years? Yes. In New Zealand, babies' diets were recorded during the first year of life. Then those babies were studied later from the ages of 8 to 18 years of age with respect to their academic abilities. Over 1000 youngsters were analyzed by standardized tests, teacher ratings, and academic outcome in high school. The conclusion was that breastfeeding played a significant rule in the outcome and that those who were breastfed longer had the best results academically. "The particular significance of the present findings is that they show the cognitive benefits that are associated with breastfeeding are unlikely to be short-lived and appear to persist until at least young adulthood."[19]

Because of the new interest (in 1997) in the effects of nurturing and breastmilk upon the brain, *Newsweek* published, as they called it, a "special edition on the critical first three years of life." In that issue Dr. Lawrence Gartner of the American Academy of Pediatrics and head of the working group on breastfeeding said: "It's hard to come out and say, 'Your baby is going to be stupider or sicker if you don't breastfeed,' but that's what the literature says."[20] Please note. He did not say that the bottlefed baby would be sick or stupid. He used only a comparative form of those words in language designed to make a point: Everything else being equal, your breast-fed baby will be healthier and smarter than if not breastfed. Dr. Michael Georgieff, a University of Minnesota professor of pediatrics and child development, wants to get more mothers to breastfeed: "If I could change one thing in society, it would be to get people to breastfeed. Breastmilk is a heck of a lot more complicated with a lot more factors that influence brain growth than cow's milk."[21]

Availability, responsiveness, and sensitivity

Mothers do need to be there with their babies and small children. William Gairdner in his book, *The War Against the Family*,[22] pointed out that three separate research studies conducted at three different major universities all clearly showed that what babies and young children need is 1) mother's availability, 2) mother's responsiveness to her child's need for comfort and protection, and 3) mother's sensitivity to her child's signals. In other words, the mother has to be there, she has to read the signals of her baby, and she has to respond to her baby in a sensitive manner. Gairdner claims that there is unanimity on this important point: "***poorly attached children are sociopaths in the making.***" To avoid poorly attached children, the answer is good mothering. The key words to good mothering, then, are these: availability, responsiveness, and sensitivity. Gairdner also states that "young children need an uninterrupted, intimate, and continuous connection with their mothers, especially in the very early months and years." With prolonged breastfeeding, the mother has an uninterrupted and continuous relationship with her baby and it's an intimate relationship as well.

Older children likewise need the presence of a parent in the home, and this includes teen-agers, a group who are prone to get into trouble when both parents are working and not at home. One mother wrote of her fears of staying home alone as a child because her mother worked. She also said she had no one to show an interest in her as a child and to be a champion for her when she needed one. In her eyes, mothering is "the most important job... that literally saves lives." As she said, "I would live in a dirt shack before I would not be there for my kids."[23]

In the fall of 1997 there was another series of studies dealing with maternal deprivation. At the Society of Neuroscience meeting in New Orleans, it was reported that children need lots of hugs and physical reassurance for proper development of the brain. Romanian children raised without this physical contact from their mother had abnormally high levels of stress hormones. This parental neglect can have lifelong consequences. "Scientists have known for decades that maternal deprivation can mark children for life with serious behavioral problems, leaving them withdrawn, apathetic, slow to learn, and prone to chronic illness... Moreover, new animal research reveals that without the attention of a loving caregiver early in life, some of an infant's brain cells simply commit suicide."[24] Does this apply to humans? Mark Smith, a psychologist at the DuPont Merck Research Labs in Wilmington, Delaware said: "These cells are committing suicide. Let this be a warning to us humans. The effects of maternal deprivation may be much more profound than we had imagined."[25] And again, in the *Newsweek* special issue on the child, it was pointed out that what makes a child unique is his experiences during the first three years of life and that physical reassurances such as cuddling and rocking stimulate brain growth and show a baby that he is loved and valued.[26]

How does stress affect the child's brain? How does a mother's presence protect or minimize the effects of stress upon her baby's brain? What researchers have learned is that stress harms brain cells of infants. During stress the body secretes large doses of cortisol to provide strength. However, cortisol can also shrink the hippocampus, the part of the brain responsible for learning, and can stunt the brain cells' ability to communicate with each other by causing the connecting dendrites to atrophy. This helps to explain why cortisol is associated with severely delayed development. That's the bad news. The good news is that the mother's physical contact with her baby protects the baby against these harmful effects.

Sometimes the importance of those first three years comes up unexpectedly. I happened to read an article on the "Big Bad Bully,"[27] behavior which is becoming quite common in schools and which is commonly ignored by teachers. The victims suffer physical or verbal abuse, continued social persecution, or rejection. What the researchers found out to their surprise was that they were studying younger and younger age groups for the cause of the bullying. First, they studied aggression in adult criminals, then adolescents, then younger children, and then two year olds! As one researcher said, "If you had told me I was going to be studying two year olds, I would have said you were crazy." The researchers discovered that bullies are made, not born; that bullies are formed "by parental behavior or by neglect" and it "begins in the early caregiver/child interaction."

Dr. Ken Magid, a clinical psychologist for twenty years, said that "second to killing someone, isolation is the worst thing we can do" and that babies should be nursed, rocked, swayed, and held. Nurturing is the key to a good outcome for your child, and it begins by "being wanted" as an infant, and "being wanted" starts at the breast of the mother, according to Magid. High-risk children have experienced trauma in their lives, and it usually happens during the first year and a half of life. The trauma is due to severe stress, said Magid, and these high-risk kids place little value on their lives and no value on other people's lives.[28]

While it is a trend for mothers to be employed outside the home, reports show that many of these mothers are not working to escape poverty.[29] One survey was of particular interest to me. Around Mother's Day in 1997, three out of four working mothers said they would still work even if they had a choice.[30] In other words, 75% of the surveyed working mothers said they would prefer to have other people raise their children for the big majority of the child's weekday waking hours.

Furthermore, working mothers often do not consider all their out-of-pocket expenses. One professor, Edward J. McCaffery at the University of Southern California and California Institute of Technology, calculated that a working mother earning $40,000 annually could end up with only $1,000 at the end of the year after deducting all expenses, taxes, and additional costs such as eating out more due to time constraints.[31] Another financial planner, Jonathan Pond, estimated that only 20% of the second income will be left over. One woman who earned $500 a week said to Mr. Pond: "By your formula, I'm only earning $100 a week. What you are telling me is that, at the end of the day I have gone absolutely nuts and am exhausted and all I have is $20 to show for it?"[32]

Are there any practical conclusions we can draw from this body of expert opinion and scientific evidence? It seems to me that all of this is clearly saying that couples need to respect the natural order and have the mother stay at home with their young children. Only a mother has the God-given ability to nourish and nurture at the breast.

A second conclusion is that couples who want to have a stay-at-home, full-time mother for their children need to make that choice well before the children arrive. That is, they need to make choices based on living on the husband's income. Some women object, "I can make more money than my husband, so he will stay home while I work." To repeat, only a mother has the God-given ability to breastfeed. I could have made three times what my husband made during the first ten years of our marriage, but we learned to live simply on his income. It wasn't until our fifth year of marriage that we bought a small home; two years later with three children we had to rent an apartment for one year. Then we went back to home ownership with the next move. I bring this up because many couples feel they have to buy a home right away. Our lifestyle was very simple, my husband's salary was well below average, but we never went hungry or went without anything we really needed. And my husband has always appreciated the fact that his wife does not have expensive tastes!

Andrew Payton Thomas in his book, *Crime and the Sacking of America,* says that children are neglected so that adults can have bigger homes and better cars. He continues:

> The rise of daycare in modern America says some painful things about us as parents and as a nation and culture, things that are easier for adults to leave unsaid. But the truth is always worth telling, and it is this: Many American parents today simply do not wish to raise their own children. Indeed, never before in history have a people become so intensely individualistic that their love for their children can be purchased so cheaply.

And what are we teaching our children? Mr. Thomas says: "Children are taught, literally from the cradle, that life is looking out for #1."[33]

Gerald Campbell, head of The Impact Group, claims that the #1 problem in our society is alienation, an emptiness, "an aloneness that cannot be tolerated by the human heart." What people really need in his estimation are "love, understanding, mercy and compassion, and commitment" from **one** person who learns to give of self "without any conditions or expectations whatsoever." He speaks of daycare as the ill of the future, and he stresses the value of a mother's presence.[34] If the child lacks "an other" or the mother, Campbell says, "eventually the child will become fearful of *all* others and, driven by rejection into an egocentric existence, will succumb to a hedonistic and utilitarian self-indulgence whose emptiness can only be a lifelong burden."[35]

To prevent alienation in our society and to develop healthy individuals who feel loved and valued, proper care during the first three years of life is crucial. Here I have tried to show the influence of nurturing and of breastmilk upon the child during the early years. What is so important about the breast-feeding — especially ecological breastfeeding and prolonged lactation — is that it gives a baby both the nurturing and the best nutrition. Prolonged lactation naturally provides those two realities that make such a positive difference! And, most importantly, prolonged lactation keeps the mother available and hopefully responsive and sensitive to her baby's needs during those crucial first three years of life.

[1] Burton White, *The First Three Years of Life*, Englewood Cliffs: Prentice-Hall, 1975.

[2] John Bowlby, *Child Care and the Growth of Love*, Baltimore: Penguin Books, 1953.

[3] Maria Montessori, *The Absorbent Mind*, New York: Dell, 1967.

[4] Selma Fraiberg, *Every Child's Birthright*, New York: Basic Books, 1977.

[5] Edgar Draper, "Potency of the Mother-Child Relationship," La Leche League Int. Conference, 1981.

[6] William and Wendy Dreskin, *The Day Care Decision*, New York: M. Evans and Co., 1983.

[7] Theodore Hellbrügge, "Early Social Development and Proficiency in Later Life," *Child and Family*, 18:1979.

[8] Hugh Riordan, "Parent-Reported Effects of Frequent Mother-Baby Separation," La Leche League Int. Conference, 1983.

[9] Ronald Lindsey, "Sexual Abuse of Children Draws Experts' Increasing Concern Nationwide," *The New York Times,* April 4, 1984.

[10] Dorothy Briggs, *Your Child's Self-Esteem*, Garden City: Doubleday, 1975.

[11] Kathleen Parker, "Quality Time Out, More Time In," *Angus Leader* (Sioux Falls), May 11, 1997.

[12] Isabelle Fox, "The Long Term Benefits of Being There," *The Nurturing Parent*, Summer 1997.

[13] Sandra Blakeslee, "Studies Show Talking With Infants Shapes Basis of Ability to Think," *The New York Times*, April 17, 1997.

[14] Gary Weisenberger, "Spend Time Nurturing Your Children," *The Cincinnati Enquirer*, May 14, 1997.

[15] Felice Freyer, "Nun Study Offers Clues to Preventing Alzheimer's," *The Cincinnati Enquirer*, November 27, 1997.

[16] Jenny Friedman, "The First Three Years," *American Baby*, April 1998.

[17] A. Lucas et al., "Breast Milk and Subsequent Intelligence Quotient in Children Born Preterm," *The Lancet*, February 1, 1992, 261-4.

[18] E. Riva et al., "Early Breastfeeding is Linked to Higher Intelligence Quotient Scores in Dietary-Treated Phenylketonuric Children," *Acta Paediatr.*, 85:1996, 56-58.

19 L. Horwood and D. Fergusson, "Breastfeeding and Later Cognitive and Academic Outcomes," *Pediatrics*, January 1988.

20 Daniel Glick, "Rooting for Intelligence," *Newsweek Special Issue*, Spring/Summer 1997, 32.

21 S. Schmickle and H. Cummins, "Nutrition Emerges as Fundamental Element of Brain Health," *Star Tribune*, June 29, 1997.

22 William Gairdner, *War Against the Family*, Toronto: Stoddart Publ., 1992.

23 C. Standley, "Letters," *The Cincinnati Enquirer*, November 11, 1997.

24 Robert Lee Hotz, "Study: Babies May Need Hugs to Develop Brain," *The Cincinnati Enquirer*, October 28, 1997.

25 Robert Boyd, "Scientists Zeroing in on Stress," *The Cincinnati Enquirer*, October 29, 1997.

26 Barbara Kantrowitz, "Off to a Good Start," *Newsweek*, Spring/Summer 1997.

27 Hara Marano, "Big Bad Bully," *Psychology Today*, September/October 1995, 50-82.

28 Ken Magid, "Nurturing Children to Become Loving Adults," La Leche League Int. Conference, 1995.

29 "Employed Women," *The Family in America Digital Archive*, January 1993.

30 Donna Abu-nsar, "Survey: Mother Was Better Mom," *The Cincinnati Enquirer*, May 9, 1997.

31 "Mom's Earnings Gobbled Up," *American Family Association Journal*, July 1997.

32 Charles Jaffe, "It May Not Pay for Both Parents to Work, Experts Say," *Washington Post*, February 13, 1994.

33 Andrew Payton Thomas, *Crime and the Sacking of America*, Washington: Brassey's, 1994.

34 Gerald Campbell, "To Heal Spiritual Alienation," Fellowship of Catholic Scholars Convention, September 20, 1997.

35 G. Campbell, personal correspondence, November 4, 1997.

13

Stepping Out with Baby

The mother of a new baby cannot simply drop out of society for two or more years. I doubt very much that the traditional African mother becomes a social recluse. The answer is as obvious as it is simple: mother takes her baby with her wherever she goes. However, such a simple solution seems to have two strikes against it. Many mothers feel culturally pressured not to bring babies with them to social gatherings; others wonder how they can take care of a nursing baby in public. The problem of nursing in public is a matter of planning and techniques that will be explained shortly, but it sometimes takes conviction, courage, and character to stand up to the pressure of one's peers.

Discreet nursing

If this is your first nursing experience, you may feel uncomfortable nursing in front of others. I certainly did! As I think back, with my first baby I always had to leave to nurse in another room — even at La Leche League meetings! There were times, however, when someone would say something positive about breastfeeding and encourage me to nurse in their presence. So I did, and I felt quite comfortable about it. As you nurse more and as your opinions and convictions about breastfeeding mature, you will find that you will be more and more comfortable with nursing outside the home.

The key to breastfeeding in the presence of people outside your immediate family is being discreet. Practice it at home, and you will soon find, as I did, that even your husband may not know you are nursing! Actually, when you wear the proper clothing, a nursing baby gives the appearance of being a sleeping baby. A mother can lift her blouse or sweater up a little from the waist and the baby's body will cover the exposed area. Knits are great for nursing since they stretch where needed. The main guideline for modest nursing is to pull your clothes up, not down. By pulling your clothes up to the nursing area, the baby covers any exposure. When you pull your clothes down to the nursing area, there is usually exposure of the breast and chest area. That type of exposure is what offends many people.

Blankets may also add to the cover-up. When wrapped around the baby, the blanket can be propped in such a way as to provide a shield of the nursing area.

Nursing can be so inconspicuous that no one has an inkling about what you are doing. There will be times when people will ask to see your nursing baby, thinking he's asleep. Your baby may be asleep, but they will not realize when asking that he is at the breast. For example, after the birth of our third baby, a friend dropped by for a visit. I was nursing at the time and continued to nurse as I answered the door. We went into the kitchen and sat at a small table to visit. Upon leaving, she asked to see the baby and was very surprised when I told her the baby was nursing. She was totally unaware of what I was doing since I had a light blanket wrapped around the baby, which provided privacy. The baby was also covering anything below the nipple area, and my clothes covered anything above. I have surprised myself at the number of places I have nursed my baby considering the fact that I once was so shy about nursing in front of others. You, too, will surprise yourself as you learn and gain confidence. The secret is to be discreet, and thus others will be more comfortable with your nursing or they simply won't know!

Many persons are very uncomfortable in the presence of a mother who nurses her baby with exposure of the breast and upper chest. There is no reason for such exposure. Baby-formula advertising materials often display exposed nursing because they want to discourage mothers from nursing. Most people are not opposed to modest nursing. For example, a friend and her young adult son dined at a local restaurant. Across the aisle was a mother nursing her baby with lots of exposure. Her son immediately requested another table and she agreed with his request. This mother is very supportive of breastfeeding. Yet she said, "It was the way she was nursing that was inappropriate. We all know that it can be done modestly."

Once you have decided you're going to take your baby with you when you go out, the rest is fairly easy. First, when nursing outside the home, it helps to have the right clothing. Two-piece outfits, dresses with hidden folds near the breast area, pant suits, ponchos, shawls or ruanas (heavy coat-length wrap-arounds with a front opening for baby that are ideal for cold climates) make nursing very easy. Never leave home, even for a short time, in an outfit that would make nursing difficult. Your baby might surprise you, and you'll find you are not prepared. A nursing baby draws less attention than a crying baby.

Another tip for modest nursing is to wear bras that have flaps which are easy to open with one hand. Since the most conspicuous part of nursing is getting ready or closing the flap, another idea is to wear a top you can't see through so a flap can remain up but unlocked. Some mothers prefer the popular stretch sports bras for nursing as they pull up easily.

In the early months, especially with your first baby, leakage can be a nuisance. The milk can wet your bra and outer clothing. This leakage can be stopped by applying pressure to the breast directly when you feel a letdown. This can be done with your hand or by folding your arms in a high position. You may use your baby for pressure on one side and your arm that's holding the baby for the other side. Sports jackets or cardigan sweaters may cover any leakage. You can also use pads when away from home. These pads can be made easily from layers of absorbent cotton cloth stitched together or by folding men's cotton handkerchiefs. Leakage is less of a problem with frequent nursing and I found it almost absent with ecological breastfeeding.

A mother may feel she has to get a baby-sitter when she goes for her first postpartum checkup. For this checkup, a baby-sitter is not necessary. Take the baby with you. Some mothers may feel comfortable nursing in the waiting room, especially if it is uncrowded or has other nursing mothers present. Others may want to make use of one of the several other rooms available in the doctor's office until they gain more confidence with public nursing.

During the early months after childbirth, it is helpful if your husband shops for groceries. To assist him, make easy shopping lists and let him do all the shopping in one store. When making the list, put the foods in the egg-milk-cheese section together, all the produce foods together and so forth. When you begin shopping, you can place the baby on your person. Many stores now have safety belts for toddlers in the seat section of the cart. When such carts are not available, back carriers for the older baby are convenient to use when shopping. Common sense tells us that a hungry baby may soon turn fussy, so it's a good idea to offer the breast in the car before taking him into a store.

When stepping out, a nursing mother may want to think ahead about certain considerations — one being the sensibilities of others, the other being her comfort when nursing. She will probably be more comfortable nursing if she is surrounded by her husband and children or people she is

111

familiar with. For example, if she is going to a meeting or a church service, she can place herself between her husband and other children; or she can sit near the wall or aisle and have her husband sit on the side where others would be seated.

In a bottlefeeding society, breastfeeding can be promoted by the example of modest nursing because such nursing can be seen as convenient and even attractive. One couple took their nursing baby to the childbirth classes that they taught while leaving their older children at home. The mothers in the class were going to bottlefeed, but some of the student-mothers changed their minds and decided to nurse their babies. The reason given was the ease with which the childbirth instructor nursed her baby and they saw how it could be done modestly.

One doesn't go against the cultural frown on public breastfeeding overnight. It takes time, and, as I've already indicated, there may be some situations — either out in public or even in your own home — in which you may want to nurse privately. Still, you will generally find that if you're quite casual, comfortable, and discreet about nursing in front of friends, they in turn will also feel comfortable.

While I was involved with ecological breastfeeding for many years, I never had a close friend who was likewise involved with this kind of mothering. I was always teaching or encouraging other parents to give it a try. Today I'm no longer nursing. Children do grow up! But we now associate with many families where extended breastfeeding is not unusual, where seeing a one or two year old at the breast is common, even a three year old occasionally. Attitudes toward the nursing mother will change as society becomes re-educated about the value of mothering and the important role that breastfeeding plays in a baby's life.

Child etiquette

The behavior of your children away from home contributes much to the happiness or unhappiness of the trip or visit and also to the impression that natural mothering makes on others. Babies have real needs to be held and to be nursed; you don't have to worry about spoiling a baby by picking him up when he cries or fusses. Children under three have very real psychological needs for mother's presence; you don't need to worry about spoiling them by bringing them along. However, taking care of these basic needs is a far cry from catering to their every desire.

For example, your child may have a favorite toy made out of metal or plastic — a great noisemaker when beaten against a wooden chair or floor. But you're taking him to church, so you substitute a soft toy instead. Speaking of taking your baby or very young child to church, attend a church service, if possible, that is more conducive to little ones. In addition to soft toys, consider bringing only those items which do not make noise, such as cloth or soft-cover books. Have your child wear soft-soled shoes. Discourage your child from playing with the hymnals in the pews since flipping the pages can produce noise and the books may drop or get torn. Again, think ahead as to what might happen. Food can be noisy and messy as well.

It might also be added that you can't expect a one- or two-year-old to sit still for 20 minutes. You expect little ones to be active. Much of the distraction comes from the parents themselves who expect their children to act like adults, and they are constantly disciplining their children. If your child is restless, carrying him or holding him on your lap may settle him. If your child is distracting to others, simply leave the pew and go to the back of church where you can hold and rock him. Don't let children run around in the back of church since this is a reward for being fussy. Sometimes a crying baby can be quieted at the breast. If the baby does not quiet down, go to the back of the church or room and hold your baby while walking back and forth; this often comforts a baby. Certainly toddlers need to be taught that church is a quiet time, but parents should realize that happy, baby sounds are not distracting to others. In fact, I miss those happy sounds in an age where most babies have pacifiers in their mouths.

The main point I want to make is this: always consider the occasion and the feelings of others who might be present. We went to a special annual banquet and were disappointed to learn that nursing babies were not allowed at the banquet. The reason given was that the previous year a mother brought her nursing baby and her baby cried the entire evening. The audience could not hear the speakers. This mother was not considerate of others, and as a result other nursing mothers were barred from future events. Nursing mothers must realize that occasionally when they attend a meeting or a talk they may have to leave the room because their baby is fussy or crying. They can return when the baby has settled down.

Natural mothering does not mean permissive mothering. When visiting other people's homes, certain courtesies should be followed, and these courtesies are taught first in your own home. Teach your children not to climb or jump or walk on furniture, teach them to eat and drink only in the kitchen or at the dining table. Don't allow them to carry a drink all around the house, and don't allow them to eat in every room of the house whether you own the house or apartment or are renting. Children need to know their boundaries and how to behave. Teach your children good habits in the beginning and they will be welcome in other homes. You will also have less work to do; no spills or crumbs to clean up in other areas of the house.

Another area of concern when visiting is your child's whereabouts. Some children stay close to mom; others tend to roam. You must be responsible for your children and know at all times where they are. Children can be taught to remain in the room with you during a visit and not to wander around the house. If they want to play outside or elsewhere, they should ask. They can also learn not to ask for food when visiting, except for water. Your job is to see that your child is not starved when you arrive. Children can also be taught to play cars and dolls on the floor instead of using good furniture, such as a piano. You can also watch that your child does not break any valuable items. Some children can avoid touching nice items and others can't. Sometimes it's best to temporarily place the item out of reach of little hands and return it before you leave. Or you may ask to visit in the family room or outside where breakables are not present. Planning a visit ahead of time may make the trip enjoyable instead of one of frustration. With natural mothering, discipline comes easily since you are always with your child and you know how he will behave. Generally, with natural mothering your outings go well.

I always made it a point to compliment my small children when we made any kind of a trip. Occasionally, there may be a visit when everything goes wrong. If this happens, try to find something positive to say to your child if you can. If you can't compliment him, review the visit with him. Let your child know why you want him to act in a certain way, how his behavior affects you or others, and how much it means to you to have him come with you. Promise him a trip to the park if he improves on the next visit. A trip to the market can be rewarded with their choice of a fruit or vegetable, something they should be eating anyway. Most little ones do like to take trips with their mother, and for most, verbal praise is sufficient.

Social life

In our society childcare is a controversial subject, and unfortunately many mothers who believe in what they are doing have been hurt by many unkind remarks. Some mothers have told me that they lost their best friends because of their differences with regard to childcare. The mother who takes her baby with her to various places and social gatherings still stands out as being different. The baby's presence says something about the mother's ideas about childcare. Peer parents who have left their babies with babysitters may be prone to make judgments, and self-justification may result in negative attitudes or judgments toward the mother-with-baby. Imagine the various currents and countercurrents when Couple A brings their baby to an evening social at Couple B's house, only to find that Couple B have sent their children elsewhere to get them out of the house for the evening! John and I were in Couple A's shoes once.

As the baby gets older, it gets even harder. As one friend said, "You only accept certain invitations, those where you know the older baby is welcome. But even when the baby is welcome, you know that the couples are wondering why you brought the baby, especially when he slept the whole time you were there. Yet, if the baby woke, I know how much he would need me."

Be proud that you enjoy being with your baby and enjoy taking him places. You will find mothers complimenting you and saying, "What a good baby! Is he that good all the time?" As another friend said, "I hear these remarks so often when I go places with my baby that I begin to wonder if other babies are all bad." You will also hear favorable judgments from mothers who will say, "I could never take my babies [or small children] anywhere even if I wanted to." In other words, your mothering and breast-feeding helps to tell the world that maybe there is a better way to raise babies and that you don't have to be tied down while nursing! And you will learn to go places with your children.

What about anniversaries and other special events? I have known several couples like ourselves who celebrate their anniversary by taking the baby or family along. This is quite easy, providing you pick a place that has reasonably quick service. Booths or out-of-the-way tables make it easier to nurse a young baby without being observed. A nice, dark atmosphere is not only romantic, but it might make for a more comfortable nursing situation. You may also want to select a place that has a highchair. The best advice is to feed your baby if possible before you arrive. If baby is sleepy and doesn't want to nurse, it may pay to wait until he nurses well and isn't tired before you take him out. Another option is to order a meal in if you feel going out to eat is too much of a hassle.

One couple turned down various business social functions and free cruises because their baby was not welcome. There was one dinner held in their honor that they could not turn down. They wrestled with the problem and found an easy solution. They hired a babysitter who came with them to hold and watch the baby in the lobby area of the restaurant. Before the dinner the mother nursed the baby well. The couple had a delightful dinner and they were at ease knowing that mom was available if needed. The baby became the star attraction with the employees so the couple was informed regularly that the baby was doing very well.

John and I have attended business socials with our baby on my back. We like the outdoors and have hiked trails while I was nursing a baby. At the beach a mother can throw a towel over her shoulder for modest nursing. Camping is so easy with a breastfed baby. When it comes to family outings, it would be hard to find a better traveler. By age three months, one of our babies had been on two overnight camping trips in a tent, a trip to the zoo, a week's trip to visit relatives, and two trips to the doctors, and there were many quick trips to the beach, picnics at the park, and a nearby wading pool. When traveling to other countries, there is no concern about the water supply, and couples claim that when flying great distances by plane, a breastfed baby requires very little attention.

The portability of breastfed babies makes them very adaptable toward a social life for the parents, but some activities are much easier than others. I would scarcely recommend taking a breastfed baby to a symphony concert at a music hall — though I know music-minded couples who have done so without a problem at concerts on university campuses. In our town babies are seen at a movie theater where old movies are shown, and there are outdoor performances of classical music and family-type music where families bring food, blankets, and chairs plus babies and young children as well.

There will be some occasions where a couple knows that their baby will not be welcome, and it would seem best to try to avoid such situations.

115

However, avoid using breastfeeding as an excuse to avoid gatherings or events that you really weren't interested in attending anyway. It may be an easy excuse, but it certainly doesn't do much to promote the idea of the real freedom of movement that the breastfeeding mother enjoys. If you wonder if you should decline an invitation because you feel that the baby might be unwelcome, why not just ask if the baby is invited too? Then explain that you are limiting your social life for a while to those occasions when you can bring your baby.

The best solution for a social life is to find those couples who accept your parenting style or who also wish to get together and bring their children. Some couples prefer to have their little ones with them and like not having to hire a babysitter. Most social situations can include your baby or older nursing child with planning and especially with like-minded friends.

Volunteering

Breastfeeding is very conducive to volunteer work in many different ways. For example, you can teach natural family planning classes or breastfeeding classes and both may entail teaching as little as one night a month.

You can provide a variety of other services without leaving your small children home. Some of these experiences can be enriching for your children as well as for yourself. When our first two children were respectively two years old and three months old, I helped "pattern" a young girl, Debbie, one day a week. Our oldest child eventually became friends with Debbie, and about a year later Debbie was allowed to spend time at our home.

When one daughter was three years old, the local Catholic grade school needed a teacher to cover topics on dating, marriage, and family for two classes, one for seventh grade girls and another for eighth grade girls. No one else would do it, so I agreed to help. My two older children were in school during the time of the classes, so I took our three-year-old with me. She had a school bag of materials to play school with, and she loved the attention from the older girls. Needless to say, I covered topics such as childbirth, breastfeeding and mothering. My daughter's only concern was that I would tell the girls that she was still nursing! There were a few times where she got tired and fell asleep in my arms, but overall she enjoyed the two classes once a week as much as I did, and she especially liked eating lunch between classes in the teachers' lounge.

When our family was young, several times I taught dental hygiene to a class of small children. These sessions were no more than 30 minutes and I always took my children with me.

Volunteer work should not be time consuming for a nursing mother, but a brief outing can be enjoyable for you and your small children. Maybe you have an elderly lady on the block who would enjoy a visit once or twice a month. Maybe you have some talent to share. One friend of mine wanted to work at the school library but would only do so if her preschooler could come with her. The school had never had this request before but consented, and the arrangement worked out well for both parties. The little girl enjoyed watching the older children use the library and was thrilled to have so many books at her disposal. One last point: be sure to tell your children how much you enjoyed having them with you and compliment them on their good behavior after your volunteer work is done.

Hospitalization

Nursing your baby away from home can occur during hospitalization of either mother or baby, but it is usually easier when it's the baby who is hospitalized. Usually obstacles can be overcome and you can bring whatever you need to make your baby's stay more comfortable. One mother who found herself in this unavoidable situation said she headed to the hospital with "rattles, mobiles, toys, tape player and a determination to nurse a baby in traction" for two weeks and then through recovery from surgery. She found that adding a few props and pillows made it easier to lean over the crib to nurse; the hardest part she found was the long nursing in the evening because it was hard on her neck. Their two other children were cared for by her husband's family while her husband was working.

Today many hospitals are willing to make arrangements in order to keep mother and baby together. The trick is to be insistent; in difficult situations it is often the assertive parents who get their way. A friend who gave birth was informed by her chiropractor after many treatments and tests that she would have to have back surgery to repair a disk. Her immediate concern was keeping her baby with her during recuperation. Her good fortune was this: 1) The hospital agreed to let the baby and father remain in her room during her entire stay. 2) Her parents took over the care of the other three children in the absence of both parents. As I have said once and I'll say again, obstacles in difficult situations can usually be overcome so mother and baby can stay together. In both cases cited, the mother-baby closeness was maintained because of the husband's strong support, the support of family and friends, and the cooperation of the hospital. Compared to the 1960s, today's hospitals are generally more open to family-centered care, and their staffs are more likely to recognize the importance of breastfeeding and the mother-infant bond.

Saying "No"

The full-time nursing mother has to learn to say no. Because she is home while so many of her contemporaries are working outside the home, she can expect to be asked to volunteer for just about everything, and she may be asked to care for other children and babies as well. She has to become discriminating, to learn the fine art of saying no without offending people. You can politely decline some jobs because they would require too much time or would be difficult to do with your baby or other children. You may decline other requests because you already have prior commitments. The one point I am making is that you will have to keep in mind the priorities of your baby and the rest of your family. Excess activity will mean excess fatigue, and excess fatigue is something you don't need. It can also be a big factor in the early return of fertility. If you want an easy way to say "no," simply say, "Sorry, I already have other plans." No one needs to know that your plans are to stay home! Learning to say no graciously is part of natural mothering.

Parental responsibility

In all of this we have seen that breastfeeding and natural mothering do not confine a mother to the house or eliminate her social life. This is not to say that natural mothering does not make its special demands. Parents are mistaken when they try to act as if they weren't parents. The couples who continue to go away on weekends without the baby or other children or who keep up other lifestyles that consistently separate them from the baby or other children for long periods of time seem to forget that parenthood carries with it a new dimension — greater responsibilities and greater joys. This change can be compared to the change from the single life to the married life. There are more responsibilities, more adjustments, and hopefully more joys to be shared. The husband or wife who acts as if he or she was still single or who does as he or she pleases without consideration for his or her spouse in marriage is immature. The parents who act without due consideration toward their new baby are likewise immature. On the other hand, the couple who choose breastfeeding and natural mothering are showing a certain sense of responsibility toward the baby by trying to do what is best for him even when it causes certain changes in their own lives.

For many couples, the occasional social restrictions of breastfeeding may be a long term blessing in disguise. Could it be that the abrupt severing of the physical relationship between mother and baby so common today hinders the baby's future development? The infant needs the loving presence of his mother, and this presence may sometimes entail her absence from a social event. If, however, the "presence demands" of breastfeeding are the occasion of providing a sounder psychological beginning for the infant, then what at first glance seems to be an infringement upon the parents' social life may very well turn out to be a distinct advantage for the child in terms of his later social life.

Breastfeeding may also help the parents to develop early the habit of thinking in terms of what is best for their family. In later years, for example, parents may find that staying home is again what is best for their teenager. Parents today complain that they don't know where their children are. As a matter of fact, some children are concerned because they don't know where their parents are! Might ecological breastfeeding teach parents something of the value of staying home with their children and making the house a home by their presence?

In summary, the ecology of breastfeeding calls for that oneness of mother and baby that we call natural mothering. Separations interfere with this. The mother has to be present to meet the various needs of her baby, and her continuous presence is the key to the natural mothering program and the maintenance of postpartum infertility. Thus, it is best for a mother to follow the practice of the typical African mother mentioned in Chapter 8. For the first 12 to 15 months the mother and baby should be practically inseparable. Baby goes where mother goes.

14

Nursing the Older Child

How long should I nurse?

Are there any guidelines to help mothers decide "How long should I nurse?" While the nursing mother's attitude about breastfeeding and about the duration of breastfeeding may change, most mothers still have some idea as to how long they want to nurse. For American mothers, the most appealing guideline might be that of the American Academy of Pediatrics.

> Exclusive breastfeeding is ideal nutrition and sufficient to support growth and development for approximately the first 6 months after birth... It is recommended that breastfeeding continue for at least 12 months, and thereafter for as long as mutually desired.[1]

In a 1990 document, UNICEF urged "all women exclusively to breast-feed their children for four to six months and to continue breastfeeding, with complementary food, well into the second year."[2] By 1994, UNICEF and the World Health Organization said:

> About six months of exclusive breastfeeding is encouraged, not four-to-six as previously recommended. Breastfeeding with complementary foods continues from six months to two years.[3]

In May of 1995 the Pontifical Academy of Sciences and the Royal Society of Great Britain co-sponsored a scientific breastfeeding conference at the Vatican. Pope John Paul II recalled that Pope Pius XII in 1941 had urged every mother to breastfeed her baby if at all possible. Pope John Paul also spoke of the many benefits of breastfeeding, endorsed the UNICEF recommendations, and asked governments to set policy which would enable women to breastfeed "up to the second year of life or beyond."[4]

Because of the Pope's endorsement of UNICEF recommendations, I reviewed UNICEF's web page on breastfeeding. In general, UNICEF has some very specific guidelines. They are given below:

"Breastmilk is the best possible food and drink for a baby. No other food or drink is needed for about the first six months of life."

"Babies should start to breastfeed as soon as possible after birth. Virtually every mother can breastfeed her baby."

"A baby needs to nurse frequently at the breast so that enough breastmilk is produced to meet the baby's needs."

"Crying… normally means that the baby needs to be held and cuddled more. Some babies need to suck the breast simply for comfort. If the baby is hungry, more sucking will produce more breastmilk."

"Mothers need to be reassured that they can feed their young babies properly with *breastmilk alone.*" (UNICEF emphasis)

"Breastfeeding should continue well into the second year of life — and for longer if possible."

UNICEF says that exclusive breastfeeding is 98% effective in avoiding pregnancy during the first six months postpartum if the mother remains in amenorrhea, and that this depends on the mother breastfeeding "frequently, day and night." Interestingly, UNICEF also recommends rest for the nursing mother and comes close to my recommendation that a mother sleep with her nursing baby while the mother takes a daily nap.

> Breastfeeding can be an opportunity for a mother to take a few minutes of much-needed rest. Husbands or other family members can help by encouraging the mother to lie down, in peace and quiet, while she breastfeeds her baby.[5]

The mother today has many options. She can set her goal for one year or for two years. She can wait and see how she feels about breastfeeding. If she chooses to nurse longer than six months or one year, she will have support from these sources. A working mother may choose to exclusively breastfeed for four months or even six months as a result of these endorsements. Many working mothers nurse their babies on weekends, all through the night in their bed, before going to work, and after returning from work. Many of these mothers only have to pump well once on their lunch break. Hopefully, even working mothers will receive support in their efforts to nurse their babies as a result of these endorsements. Such support is available that wasn't available prior to the 90s.

Nature's norm

Experience has shown that the mother who follows this book's pattern of natural mothering will usually be nursing well beyond her baby's first birthday. In our last survey of breastfeeding and amenorrhea, the group that followed this pattern averaged 14.5 months of amenorrhea and averaged almost 26 months of breastfeeding. Over 45% of the 98 mothers who were involved in ecological breastfeeding nursed beyond the child's second birthday and 17 of the 98 mothers nursed for three years or more. Thus it is evident that some normal American women are experiencing the same kind of extended natural mothering pattern that is common in cultures that are very much in touch with nature. In this chapter we will use the term "older child" to refer to the baby who has passed his first birthday, and we'll be looking at some reasons for nursing the older child, some cultural attitudes, and some ways for the long-term nursing mother to find support when some of the other women tell her she's crazy.

Weaning frequently occurs when babies are 9 or 10 months old. In our first survey, out of the entire group, 25.0 percent of mothers weaned between 9 and 12 months (the most common time in our survey), and 20.6 percent weaned between 13 and 16 months (the next most common time.) This, keep in mind, was from a group of women interested enough in breastfeeding to have read the first, privately published edition of this book.

Remember that people are not used to seeing women who nurse longer than a year and most people have a very limited view of breastfeeding. Strangely, even some of those who are most adamant about breastfeeding in the early months for the full range of nutritional and emotional reasons are either shocked or surprised to learn that a mother is still nursing an older child. Then there are those who look at breastfeeding only in terms of short-term nutrition and others who see it only as a means of birth control. If you look at breastfeeding primarily or even exclusively as a way of satisfying baby's hunger pangs, then you can readily see why a baby could be weaned by 10 months. With the introduction of solids and early use of the cup, breastfeeding is no longer physically necessary for hunger satisfaction. (However, occasionally it remains physically necessary for medical reasons, e.g., allergies.) If you look upon breastfeeding primarily as a means of avoiding a pregnancy, once menstruation resumes there is no reason to continue the nursing relationship. On the other hand, if breastfeeding involves a whole method of childcare and if the breast is looked upon as a wonderful aid for mothering, then there is no need to have a cut-off date. A mother may as well take advantage of this easy form of mothering while she can. Two or three years of nursing may sound like a long time, but in terms of the child's lifetime it is brief.

Unfortunately, some people find cruel explanations for prolonged nursing. They may say that the mother is smothering the child or that she is nursing for sexual gratification. Some infer that she is using the baby as a birth-control device. They worry that the mother is being neglectful or that the baby will be psychologically damaged. Will the baby boy grow up to be effeminate or will the child have homosexual tendencies? Is the baby addicted to the breast? The above fears are unfounded. In fact, the widely publicized homosexual trends today occur in an age of bottlefeeding and early weaning practices. Certainly, prolonged breastfeeding is not accountable in our society for this incidence. In the light of the severely critical comments that are sometimes made, it is helpful to have the support of others when you are nursing the child according to his own timetable.

Nursing needs of the older child

Maria Montessori supports nature's guidelines for mothering. Her views about early infant care are well expressed in her famous book, *The Absorbent Mind*. She advises parents to respect the child's natural development. "Localized states of maturity must first be established, and the effort to force the child's natural development can only do harm. It is nature that directs. Everything depends on her and must obey her command."[6]

Once a mother has decided to go along with her baby and let him wean himself at his own pace, she may have some second thoughts. Perhaps she thought this meant a couple of extra months — and now he's almost two. Could he possibly still have a need for breastfeeding? Interestingly enough, we see nothing strange when a two-year-old uses a bottle or a pacifier. However, because the long-term nursing mother is an exception in our culture, the doubts persist. She can take comfort in these passages from Eda LeShan's *How Do Your Children Grow?*

> We also have to understand, and this holds true all through parenthood, that when a need is met, it goes away. Children of any age do not continue to behave in certain ways unless there is a need. When they are finished with it, they will give it up. Sometimes it may go on longer than we expect, and a parent will worry because a 16-month-old is still nursing. This is a very natural tendency. We think the things that are happening will go on forever. The truth is that they will go on only as they are needed.[7]

However, we worry far too much about the need lasting too long. Satisfying a legitimate need is less likely to do any damage than the opposite, cutting off that satisfaction too quickly. The one thing that upsets parents and children more than anything else is the unfinished business of any one phase of life. If a child needs to go through some kind of an emotional experience, and he doesn't go through it at the time that is most appropriate, it is never finished, according to LeShan.[8]

Prolonged breastfeeding may also prove helpful in emergency situations or during an illness. Temporary emergency situations, such as car trouble or bad weather conditions, may cause a period of isolation during which nursing can be advantageous. Prolonged breastfeeding may influence your baby's health even after his first birthday. The older baby who loses his appetite during an illness will usually take some nourishment from the breast at a time when he might not take any other foods. Here is a story of one mother who was grateful that she had continued to nurse her child:

> When our second son was being seen by his pediatrician for his first yearly checkup, the doctor questioned me about his still being nursed. "Aren't you ever going to wean him? You know, he's not needing this physically for nutrition anymore." I answered, "Great! I'll go home with a pacified doctor and a very frustrated baby." We both laughed and I assured the doctor that he would wean — but at **his** own rate.

Two months later the baby became ill with an intestinal virus. His fever was 105 and we rushed him to the hospital. For two days and nights he was kept on clear liquids and nursing. Even with this, the diarrhea was so severe that the doctor ordered IV's to prevent further dehydration. This lasted 48 hours. During this period I couldn't even nurse him. Actually, he was so sick that he slept most of the time — so I was the one who suffered with full breasts.

Hand expressing and pumping with the breast pump somehow just didn't seem to empty my breasts as completely as a nursing baby does. I'm certain that a good deal of it was psychological for me too. By the end of the second day the doctor asked me, "Do you think he still remembers how to nurse after this long? If he does and **since** it's breastmilk — I'll let him have the milk. I know he'll regain his strength faster. Also it won't upset his intestines like foreign milk would." Still remember how? You don't practice something several times a day for 14 months and then forget in two days! I only wish I had words to describe how eagerly he settled against me — knowing **exactly** where he was going. Joy and relief flooded us both!

Later during a visit to the doctor's office, the pediatrician gave me one of the nicest compliments I ever had with a nursing experience: "You've shown me how important it is to follow a baby-led weaning pattern, and never will I pressure a mother about weaning again."

The most common reason given for prolonged breastfeeding is the special relationship that a mother has with her child. This closeness is strengthened over a period of two or three years through the nursing relationship, and it cannot easily be lost once the breastfeeding comes to an end. The bond is still there, and a mother can maintain it through other avenues of affection and communication, physical or verbal. One wonders whether the "generation gap" begins at such an early time. Would more parents be in tune with their children if they had breastfed for a considerable length of time? Would children be more sensitive to their parents' feelings if they had experienced this long-term relationship with the one parent in early childhood?

Certainly there are other factors that can influence our relationships with our children, but today we parents need all the help we can get to do a better job of raising our children. We also need easier methods, and breastfeeding makes the job easier at least during those early years. Whether it helps in later years is speculative, but some parents have told us there is a bond and closeness with their breastfed children that they didn't achieve with their bottlefed children. This closeness has also matured them and given them a deeper appreciation of the needs of their older children and even of other children in the immediate neighborhood.

The warm relationship that develops during the first years as part of natural mothering certainly is a big help in developing open communications. I am not suggesting that the mother who lets her children breastfeed into the second, third, or fourth year will have no communication problems with them in the teen years. I am the last one to suggest that. What I am suggesting, however, is that the close relationship and the habit of being open to the young child's needs gets a parent off to a good start. The parents who work at maintaining this habit of openness to the child's needs for time and affection should have less difficulty during those adolescent years. One mother wrote:

> My second oldest child was 15 yesterday. As I look back as I have done repeatedly in the last 10 years since my joy of discovering breastfeeding, I'm still regretful about those years of bottlefeeding with my first three children. It is said that you don't cry over spilled milk, but I do, and I think that is my underlying motivation in trying to help other mothers and families.

We have all heard various psychologists say something to the effect that a child's character or the way he will respond to different situations is pretty much set by the time he is six years old. If during a good half of those years he found security and warmth at his mother's breast, as he needed it and not as someone else dictated, then this would seem to be a good foundation of trust for the later years.

Keep this in mind however: even the best childcare does not eliminate the effects of Original Sin. Genesis 4 tells us that breastfed Cain killed breastfed Abel. In other words, a long and strong breastfeeding relationship is no guarantee that problems will not develop later. Still, the relationship developed through breastfeeding may reduce the extent of later problems or help in the recovery from later problems.

Regardless of what the future holds, the fact still remains that as parents of young children we are called to respond to their needs with ourselves and not just with things that money can buy. Doing our best for the child, giving him the best of everything doesn't mean only clothes, schools, toys, lessons, transportation, vacations, tutors, babysitters, and money. Giving of ourselves to young children does not involve money or material things; it only involves our time.

In today's world of divorce, two parents working, and consumerism, parents tend to finance their children's affection. In the old days dad could stay home on the weekends, but now dad or mom are expected to entertain their child with numerous outside events that often cost money. Now some older parents are financing resort-like homes so they can lure their grown children back since they fear their children will not want to spend much time with them. This trend was well explained by Froma Harrop:

> The money-for-love arrangement has been around for a long time... Many parents seem genuinely concerned that their children, once they are grown, will have little interest in spending time with them... A couple approaching retirement explains they are building an 8,000-square-foot house to attract grown children and grandchildren... As two-income couples have less time to spend with their children, they can replace missing time with money. Parental guilt plays a part.[9]

There is no doubt that while natural mothering at times is easier than using artifacts, it does take time. Best of all, it always gives individual attention that is a wise investment in the child's future. Even Margaret Mead expressed concern over the type of care a young child receives in daycare centers: "Only individual attention can turn a child into a full human being, capable of growth." She criticized a frequent change in the mother-figure and noted that a small child "needs someone who is intensely interested in him or her, who will spend endless hours responding and initiating, repeating sounds, noting nuances of expression, reinforcing new skills, bolstering self-confidence and a sense of self." A child who receives such continuity, she claims, "can survive a great many changes of place and person later." Persons who do not have such care "have less capacity to trust the world, to leave home happily, and to form wider and more intense relationships with other people later."[10] Considering the many changes of place and persons that some children experience in our mobile society, the individual time and attention spent in natural mothering is a sound investment.

Consider another benefit of prolonged nursing that lets the child wean at his own pace. Natural breastfeeding helps parents to accept and love the child for what he is. Instead of imposing outside norms, natural mothering looks to the inner growth pattern of the child. The child's growth in all its phases is guarded and respected. These phases of growth are not forced to end too early, nor are they forced to remain when the need is no longer present. This acceptance and love for the child as he is may help the parents to accept him at his own level of interests and abilities in later years.

Another tremendous benefit from prolonged breastfeeding is the stimulation that the child receives when his mother takes him with her. He is exposed to a wide variety of social circumstances, and he has the security of his parents or his mother wherever he goes. This stimulation is far greater than that which he would receive by remaining at home with sitters.

By no means least among the benefits of prolonged nursing is the continuation of family-centerness. In the family where ecological breastfeeding is used in the first year, the baby is always a part of the family: the parents don't take off without him. Likewise when the mother continues to let her baby nurse beyond the first year, she will not be leaving him for extended periods of time. Instead, she will want to be near him, and she and her husband will plan recreational activities that are family oriented. The child who grows up in such a family today is lucky indeed. Family life in America is such that professionals are becoming concerned; it is too common for parents to look upon children as a burden or as second-class citizens within the family. There is a concern that parents too often are striving to get away from their children. The extended nursing of natural mothering is a tendency in the other direction.

Some characteristics of the older nursing child

What can you expect from the older nursing child? First, you will find that your child will ask for the breast at any time or place, especially during the first year or two of life. In fact, he may ask for it at a time when you do not want him to ask, when you are around distant relatives and new friends. Strangers present a new environment to the child, and in looking for security from his mother, he often seeks it at the breast.

You can avoid some embarrassment for yourself by having the child call the breast "ma-ma" or "mum-mum" or any word other than something like "nursie." Your child may also not call it anything; he simply informs you of his intentions by pulling or tugging or lifting up your top. If other persons are around, they will probably not pick up the clue. You may leave temporarily to nurse, or you may explain the situation, or you may tell your child "later," or you may nurse on the spot but do it in such a way as not to offend those nearby.

You will find it is harder to nurse modestly with a bigger baby. He is too big for blankets; thus the blanket can't be used as a shield. There is a good chance he will dislike clothing too close to his face. He may play with your clothing in a playful manner so that attention is actually drawn toward the nursing area. As your child gets past his second birthday, it begins to get easier. Eventually he will be willing to wait. Obviously, it is easier to nurse an older baby when you are among those who understand and appreciate this type of mothering. How a mother handles the situation will vary with the place and the age of her baby — whether he is 12 months old or two years old, but experience and conviction are the most important factors in how the mother responds.

Your older nursing child will be talkative, playful, and affectionate. His responses are greatly varied. At times he will even tell you where to nurse him! He can even be funny. There is also more give and take. He can appreciate the fact that you are busy, and he can wait a few minutes for a nursing until you finish your task. He can also learn to wait that one hour during the church service as he gets older.

You can also expect nursing sprees. Some days you will wonder why your child wants to nurse every hour for a few minutes or why the child wants to nurse almost continuously during the night. And why does he come to you for a quick nursing when he's in the middle of play with siblings and neighborhood children? We noticed, for example, that after we moved to another state our three-year-old nursed almost constantly during the night for several weeks. Sometimes increased nursing can be explained and other times it can't be explained, but trust that this too will pass in due time and the child will reduce the frequency.

As your child reaches an age between two to three years, you will find that he will not want to nurse in front of others who are strange to him. He may not want his parents or brothers or sisters to discuss his nursing with others in his presence or to tattle to his friends. His wishes should be respected within the family. As a couple who promotes breastfeeding, we still respect our children's feelings on this matter in how we answer the typical question: "How long did you nurse?" Many times we tell the numbers. At other times we speak in generalities, such as the time we were asked at a university where our child was attending and was fairly well known.

You may also find your child is still nursing frequently in spite of being older. In writing and talking with other mothers, I find that it is common for older children reaching their second or even third birthday to be still nursing quite frequently. Some people feel that if a child has other brothers or sisters to keep him busy, or if the mother keeps her child interested in other activities, the child will lose interest in the breast. I find little support for this view. In the busiest of households and with mothers who stimulate their youngsters toward various interests and activities, the child will still take the time to nurse in the midst of it all.

Night feedings can be expected while your older child is still nursing. In our study of mothers who nursed in a manner similar to the natural mothering program, most mothers gave night feedings for as many months as they nursed, averaging approximately 24 months of night feedings. Usually the last feedings to be dropped are those related to sleep. Therefore, toward the end of his nursing career the child may be nursing only before naptime or before bedtime in the evening. When this situation happens, then no one except your husband will know that your child is still nursing — unless you tell them.

Separations

An older nursing baby can begin to take brief separations from mom, such as an hour or two at the most, especially if he is having a good time at home or if he likes his caregiver. These brief separations can begin sometime after the child's first birthday, but the time varies when a child accepts these separations of an hour or two willingly.

Children find it easier to accept separations of one or two hours during the daytime and early evening than at night. Upon your return you may find the babysitter or your husband or your older children telling you that your child was just beginning to miss you and was asking about you. Our last two children experienced their first separation of about one and a half hours at 15 and 18 months respectively. The occasion was their parents' decision to have dinner out alone but close to home. The 15-month-old started missing me before I returned; the 18 month old hardly knew I left. When I left the latter child the first time for a full day at a local conference, he was five and showed no signs of distress that day. However, for the next few days he would not let me out of his sight.

I don't want mothers to set any goals by my babies, nor do I want to have mothers feel guilty for leaving their children at home. I mention this only because I've learned of mothers who misinterpreted what I've written elsewhere and felt guilty because they left a two-year-old at home for a short time. You and your child can communicate and work these things out together. If you try a brief separation sometime and it doesn't work, then wait a while before you try again. Once separations do begin, they should be infrequent at first with a lot of consideration given to the child and his reaction to any separation.

Nighttime separations can be much harder for a child under two years of age. A child who has been nursed as described in this book may at 18 months choose to stay home with dad while mother runs to the store during the daytime. But this same child may have a strong need to be near mother at night. We accepted this fact, mainly from past experiences, and took our younger children with us everywhere in the evenings (be it social, for meetings, or for classes we taught) for their first two years of life. When they turned two, after a few explanations and discussions, each child would decide if he or she was big enough to stay home for the two or three hours we would be gone. Even then, we would occasionally come home to a child staring out the window waiting for our return. Sometimes the siblings pretended they were talking to me on the phone so they could tell the youngest that mom will be home soon.

Nighttime separations are easier to handle when the older children understand the situation and are therefore very helpful or the babysitter is compassionate and is willing to hold the child a lot and read to him. If one nighttime separation is hard on your child, then bring him with you the next time. That's what we did. Most two year olds soon decide that adult company and meetings are boring and decide to stay home at nights on their own.

Sometimes bringing a babysitter along with you and your child or children is a good alternative to separation. For example, when our first three children were 2, 4, and 6 years old, we played tennis at a park where the playground was across a busy street from the courts. So we could play tennis without worrying about the children, we hired a neighborhood girl they liked to come with us and watch them at the playground. This way we all had a good time.

We found a similar situation while teaching natural family planning classes with an active baby. Our fourth child was content to remain near us during our two-hour classes, but our fifth child was everywhere. So his sisters, knowing that this baby needed to be near me, took turns coming to class to watch him while we taught. This arrangement worked well for us.

Overnight and weekend separations can be hard on young children. In a question-and-answer session following a talk in Cincinnati, Dr. Marshall Klaus, co-author of *Maternal-Infant Bonding*, was asked at what age would it be all right for the parents to leave their child for a weekend or overnight trip. He advised parents to wait until the child was at least four or five years old. He also suggested calling their child each night of their absence, but I know a couple who did this and their child began to cry on the phone. So I leave this up to the parents. I still feel it is best to include little ones on your trips and vacations as I have stated before, and my husband feels just as strongly on this issue because of his regrets that his parents left him in the care of others while they took off.

In summary, there seem to be four factors related to non-traumatic separations — the age of the child, the length of the separation, the frequency of separation, and your temporary mother-substitute. Wait until your child is ready. Then by making your initial separations short, you build trust; just about the time he starts to miss you, you're home. Make your separations infrequent; children generally do not like their parents — especially both parents—out of the home several nights a week. Finally choose someone close to your children to be there for them in your absence.

Final weaning

With natural mothering the time of final weaning is unpredictable because it is at the child's own pace. Sometimes a mother expects to nurse a baby for about two years only to be surprised to find that her child weans much earlier. Or a mother may decide to nurse only one year and find at three years she is still nursing! A mother who finds her baby weaning earlier than she planned must realize that mothering isn't limited to the breast, that there are other ways to meet his needs. She can still provide him with lots of love and body contact and do many things with him. She can be assured that she satisfied his needs at the breast.

Don't compare your breastfeeding or your mothering to somebody else. We want to avoid competitive mothering. The main point is to remember to enjoy your baby at every stage and at *his* schedule. Contented mothering is that geared to our baby.

The example of others

The desire to nurse an older baby often comes by way of example. A mother can be encouraged to continue nursing her child if she knows another mother who is nursing an older baby. Other mothers want to nurse longer but quit because they know of no one else who is doing it. This is understandable. Despite many benefits that mothers find with the extended nursing of natural mothering, it is still a difficult thing to consider in a bottlefeeding culture. Most people do not appreciate long-term nursing unless they have done it, have known a close friend or relative who has done it, or find themselves in the situation where it is evident that their baby still desires to be at the breast.

Your own feelings about nursing the older child will change as your nursing experience develops or matures with the age of your baby. Intellectual reasons for prolonged lactation will probably play a small part in this change of attitudes. What will change your feelings on the subject at the time will be that one-year-old or two-year-old in your arms who still needs you. The pressure from society to wean may encourage you to stall a feeding only to find tears rolling down your child's cheeks — and you lovingly take him to breast. Secondly, the relationship is too enjoyable for its ending to be hastened, something which is hard for many to understand in a society where many nursing mothers quit in the first months of life.

Long-term nursing in a bottlefeeding culture

How can you handle the reaction of others to long-term nursing? First of all, you can appreciate why others feel the way they do about prolonged nursing when you try to picture somebody else's two or three year old still nursing. I have nursed an older child, yet it's always a surprise to hear that another older child is still nursing when you see how big he is. Having been there, I can appreciate how others feel about long-term nursing because many parents have not had this experience. What makes the difference in your feelings about nursing your older child is the fact that this child is *your* child.

The number of mothers who are experiencing long-term nursing is gradually increasing. But because this practice is not common in a bottlefeeding culture, people can have unfavorable reactions. Some are simply amazed to learn that a mother could still be producing milk two or three years after childbirth. Because your audience may think you're crazy, there is no reason in the world why you would have to volunteer the information.

If a situation develops where you find you have to tell, my husband and I have found that the best policy in handling other persons' questions is usually to be honest and "sure-headed," not apologetic. You will discover that there is very little static or none at all when you convey the attitude that you are confident in what you are doing and that you feel that this is the way it should be done. If you don't like to give personal reasons, you can always refer to women in other parts of the world and to those American women who nursed for several years before the "bottle" generations. Some parents can mention health reasons. Some mothers may find it helpful to throw the attention to another nursing mother by saying, "I have a friend who is nursing a child who is even older than ours." If you personally know of someone who is nursing a child older than yours, you will find that this offers you a great deal of support. If you don't, think of me as your "friend." I nursed my last three children for four, five, and five years.

The best support a nursing mother can have, however, is her husband. If her husband is 100% behind her, then an unkind remark will not hurt nearly as badly. It is wonderful to have a husband step in and handle the discussion, especially when the reactions are quite strong and negative.

In the last analysis, if you do prolonged nursing because your child still wants to nurse and not out of some personal whim "to show the world" or to compete with somebody else, if you recognize that this is common in many cultures of the world, and if your husband supports you, then you have nothing to fear. On the other hand, you should not look down on the mother who gives the childcare typical of our bottlefeeding culture. Ignorance is usually the greatest barrier to freedom. A person can't choose something before she knows about it, and many mothers have never been exposed to natural mothering.

Today we hear much talk about changing life styles, some of which concerns a return to nature. This doesn't mean that we have to move out of the city or that everybody has to have an organic garden. Nature isn't to be found just in the fields and the forest or among the animals. Though our nature is incomparably higher and more complex than that of the animal and vegetable kingdoms, we still have a nature and we are better off when we live according to it instead of going against it.

Obviously there are different degrees of living with or going against our common human nature. I think that almost everyone would agree that the parents who killed their child would be going against our human nature in a most serious way; the same would be said about parents who abused their child by beating him or by neglecting him. I would like to suggest that there are more subtle ways of going against our human nature, or at least of not living in accord with it, and that this is particularly true in a culture that is fascinated by technology and "being modern." That fascination brought in the bottle and almost eliminated breastfeeding. Fortunately, there are an increasing number of people who recognize the wisdom of fostering the natural, and breastfeeding has made a significant comeback.

What we need is a lifestyle that incorporates a new respect for living in full accord with our human nature. For the present, this will also demand a new independence from the dictates of our bottlefeeding culture. Such a lifestyle would support the close ties between mother and baby for as long as the child's needs keep him nursing. Since our present Western culture doesn't support such a lifestyle, it is all the more important for every nursing mother to have loving support from her husband. When he is with you emotionally on this issue, it matters little what others may think.

On the other hand, if a husband is indifferent or even hostile to the idea of breastfeeding and prolonged nursing, then other support may be in vain. Therefore it is extremely important that a nursing mother be a wife who communicates well with her husband. She should share not only her conclusions but likewise her reasons and the materials that she has found helpful and convincing. Many husbands will have open (or at least secret) admiration for a wife's ability to make an intelligent case for extended nursing. Others will give their support if they see that the wife herself is really convinced and wants her husband's support regardless of how good a case she makes. What is important is that the husband be proud of his wife's willingness and desire to take care of their baby's needs in this way so that his wife will find the strength to persevere in the face of cultural customs.

The strongest case for natural mothering and prolonged nursing is made by mothers who have raised one baby by cultural standards and then later raised one by natural mothering. Repeatedly, those who changed their attitudes and tried prolonged breastfeeding have found it to be a rewarding experience. It has been common for them to state that they wished they had nursed previous children in a similar manner and that they feel mothers are missing out on a valuable experience by weaning too early.

Natural child spacing

There is no way to predict how long a mother will nurse. There is no way to predict the length of amenorrhea for any particular woman. The late return of fertility and menstruation will happen usually in those women who let their babies nurse frequently during the day, without restriction during the daily nap, and during the night. Some women have a body chemistry that is more favorable to a later return, but the majority of women need a lot of stimulation to hold back menstruation. That's another reason why natural mothering is so helpful. Remember that the women who followed closely the guidelines of natural mothering experienced their first period on average between 14 and 15 months postpartum. Obviously, this length of amenorrhea was possible only because of nursing an older child.

[1] American Academy of Pediatrics, *Pediatrics*, December 1997.

[2] UNICEF, *Children and Development in the 1990s*, World Summit for Children, New York, September 29-30, 1990.

[3] UNICEF/WHO, "Infant and Young Child Nutrition," 47th World Health Assembly, May 1994.

[4] Pope John Paul II, *L'Osservatore Romano*, May 24, 1995.

[5] UNICEF, "Breastfeeding," www.unicef.org, May 18, 1999. For current information, refer to this web page.

[6] Maria Montessori, *The Absorbent Mind*, New York: Dell, 1967.

[7] Eda LeShan, *How Do Your Children Grow?*, New York: David McKay, 1972.

[8] Ibid.

[9] Froma Harrop, "Parents Finance Kids' Affection," *The Cincinnati Enquirer*, January 3, 1998.

[10] Margaret Mead, "Working Mothers and Their Children," *Catholic World*, November 1970, 78.

15

To Husbands

By John F. Kippley

If you are a typical husband, you may not share your wife's enthusiasm for reading books and other literature about breastfeeding. Perhaps your wife has given you this chapter and asked you to read it, so I'll make it brief. I'm just going to share a few thoughts that you might find helpful.

First of all, you can be proud of your wife for breastfeeding your baby. She's doing what is best for him — and for her. Give her support because she needs it from you. She needs to know that you are grateful she's doing what is best for your baby.

Secondly, there are some experiences that you will probably miss, or at least have less of, than the fathers of bottlefed babies. Because the breastfed baby has health advantages over the bottlefed baby, your baby will most likely have fewer illnesses, allergies, and so on, than if your wife did not nurse.

You are also going to miss the experience of the horrible mess that is made when mothers (or fathers) try to feed solids to babies in the early months. I can still distinctly remember one Saturday morning back in my bachelor days when I stopped to pick up a buddy for golf. He invited me in for a cup of coffee while his wife was feeding a very young baby. The pureed baby food was all over everything — hair, face, arms, and clothes. It made an indelible impression, and it's an experience I haven't missed at all with our breastfed children. From the above, it is also obvious that you are going to miss the expenses associated with baby foods and increased medical or dental problems.

One thing we have had some questions on is the idea of the baby sleeping in bed with his parents. We have been told of husbands who initiated the idea, and we have also heard from wives telling us that they think their husbands would object to having the baby as an intruder in the marriage bed, that the presence of the baby will interfere with marital intimacy. The simple answer is that it doesn't. "Sleeping with baby" doesn't mean he's with you all the time. He will normally be asleep before you go to bed, and you can put him in another bed for a while. Or, your wife may nurse him to sleep in another bed or in the general living area and leave the baby there until you are ready to bring him to bed with you. I'm sure that any couple with a little ingenuity can have their marital intimacy and their "sleeping with baby" too.

Keep in mind that it is the baby's **regular frequent and unrestricted** suckling that brings about breastfeeding's side effect of extended natural infertility. If you train the baby to sleep by himself all through the night, your wife may very well be deprived of the suckling stimulus she needs for continued natural infertility and maybe even for her continued ample milk supply. It also helps to keep in mind that those night nursings are saving you the trouble of getting up for the middle-of-the-night bottle warmings.

Being a father calls for a little maturity. The baby is your child, and his needs call for more instant satisfaction than yours. If your wife is preparing dinner and the baby really needs to nurse, don't get upset if dinner is a few minutes late. Don't be afraid to pitch in with the dishes when your baby needs his mother. And finally, when all that your baby needs is a changing, some holding, some walking, or some rocking, be sure to get in on the act. There is something very satisfying about having your babe fall asleep in your arms.

Support your wife when she allows your child to wean at his own pace. You thought he would never talk — and then he did and won't stop. You think he's never going to wean — and he will when he's ready. In other cultures throughout the world it is common for three-year-olds to still nurse. Your child will be big and older before you know what has happened. Relax and enjoy the nursing years, and you'll be glad you did.

16

Sex and the Lactating Mother

There are individual differences with regard to the sex drive, and one's sex drive may be influenced by several factors such as alcohol, fatigue, natural hormones including those during pregnancy and lactation, or artificial hormones. Pregnancy and nursing may affect a woman's sexual drive. For those women who have no change or else find an increased desire, there is generally no problem. A few rather exceptional women find that lactation increases their sexual drive to such an extent that they experience erotic sensation when nursing. These women can accept these feelings as normal, not feel guilty or bad, and let these feelings subside naturally. Weaning the baby is not the answer. This situation is usually uncommon, but some women have been accused wrongly of nursing an older baby for their own sexual gratification.

On the other hand, women who find a reduced interest in sex while nursing may wonder if they are abnormal. One nursing mother told us she had a very strong desire to have sex with her husband during pregnancy (even prior to labor the urge was very strong), but immediately following childbirth she lost all interest in genital sex. Other women have written that while nursing they lost their desire for the genital embrace and wondered if something was wrong with them.

Some of these women have also read materials which give the impression that if you nurse, your interest in sex will increase. That can increase the worry and concern if you find that this is not your situation but that the exact opposite is true.

A decreased sex drive for the nursing mother appears to be very common. A home birth instructor who continues to have contact with nursing mothers after birth finds that almost all the breastfeeding mothers she talks to have lost their sexual drive. She claims the main reason is that the woman's body is constantly in touch with her baby and thus receives a sense of physical and emotional well-being in the motherly act of nursing. Women are cuddlers and caressers and the nursing mother derives a great deal of emotional satisfaction as her infant smiles, coos, touches her face, lips, chest and looks up into her face. These tender moments or emotional highs add to the emotional well-being of the mother.

On the other hand, hormones certainly cannot be ignored and probably play an important role in the changes which occur during these maternal times. For example, why do some women have their sexual desire heightened during pregnancy but find it almost eliminated during nursing?

There is a tremendous amount of time and energy spent in the care of a baby so fatigue can be a factor in reduced sexual feelings. I would hope fatigue would be a factor only occasionally since fatigue can be minimized if the mother is sleeping with her baby. A mother who takes time to take a nap and to enjoy her baby and the nursing times together will be more refreshed than the mother who continually tries to get something done around the house or gets too involved with outside activities. I also believe that fatigue may decrease the milk supply, reduce the strength and occurrence of the letdown, and bring an early return of menstruation.

Some remedies to physical changes that may occur in a nursing mother's body are as follows:

Dry vagina

Vaginal dryness can cause pain or discomfort, especially during the marriage act, and can be relieved by an application of a water-soluble lubricant such as KY jelly on the external lips of the vulva; KY jelly is not a contraceptive jelly. Vaseline is not water-soluble and is generally unsatisfactory as a vaginal lubricant. For a cost-free and always available lubricant, you might try your own saliva. Another readily available lubricant is raw egg white, a substance also thought to aid sperm migration.

Leaking breasts

Spraying of milk from the breasts during lovemaking is normal and should not be any concern to your husband or yourself.

Sore breasts

Some nursing mothers not only experience sore nipples but cracked and bleeding nipples as well. Obviously, at these times the breasts are temporarily untouchable, and great tenderness should be a main concern during lovemaking.

My advice based on personal experience and those of other nursing mothers is to administer treatment to the nipple area immediately once the tiniest amount of soreness is felt. Many believe that soreness is eliminated if the baby is latched on properly. Treatments involve moist or cream applications or warm air from a portable hair dryer. With the hair dryer, I found the warm, dry air gave me immediate relief.

Changes involving lovemaking

Your baby may cause a few scheduling changes. For example, if you and your husband are all ready for bed but your baby is awake and playful, be patient and enjoy your baby. The "family bed" is no real deterrent to marital intimacy because once your baby falls asleep, you may choose to place him elsewhere or go elsewhere yourselves. Because some babies tend to be very wide awake in the evening hours, sometimes parents find lovemaking more convenient in the early morning hours, lunch hour, the weekends, or baby's nap.

Even though the drive is absent, a wife can still engage in the marital embrace and enjoy lovemaking on the basis of loving and giving herself to her husband. The husband can appreciate his wife's feelings and not expect the same frequency of lovemaking nor the same strong response or the same type of foreplay from his wife since her sexual desires have changed.

Marriage will have various times of readjustments, and babies bring a new adjustment phase to marriage whether it's a first baby or a fifth baby. Parenthood brings new decisions, worries, concerns, times of happiness, and sad happenings that can influence lovemaking. Attitudes on parenting and children can affect lovemaking. The wife, for example, may talk constantly about the children when her husband is home instead of spending some time discussing his day.

Another example would be the feelings some women have with regard to childcare. Her husband is so wrapped up with his job or jobs, spends lots of time with some athletic team or hobby, or watching sport programs on the weekends, that she feels child-rearing is entirely on her shoulders. On the other hand a man may work hard to provide for his family but may not feel appreciated in his role as provider. These feelings do affect lovemaking. Both spouses need to feel loved and both need to feel appreciated.

But since we are talking about the decreased sexual interest on the part of the woman, it needs to be said that she especially needs her husband's support at this time. By his availability and his caring for her and the children, she likewise responds by loving and caring for him. I have often felt most loving toward my husband during his special caring times for our children and me. A man's caring for his wife and children naturally generates a loving wife, and a wife's care and concern for her husband helps to make him feel special.

Both partners can appreciate that nursing can be a positive time of togetherness for them. He can put his arm around her or they can share thoughts and plans for themselves and their children as she rocks and nurses the baby to sleep at night. Music, reading, prayer, or a bedtime snack are other things a couple can share as the woman nurses. Thus baby's nursing time does not mean "no husband" time. The wife may use non-nursing times to show affection also, such as a greeting kiss at the door.

Communication among caring couples helps during the readjustment periods, and that means talking about your feelings. Many problems in marriages can be avoided or reduced through adequate communication and concern for the other. Hopefully, those couples who give birth together and share in child-rearing and in natural family planning have already communicated in those areas and have found discussions related to their married life easier. Nursing is an excellent time for such discussions. Shared parenting likewise can strengthen the marriage and the family.

Values and moral principles are important, too. If husband and wife differ on values and moral principles, the marriage will not be as good even with lots of communication. Both must see that sex and marriage are so much more than genital. Their covenant for better and for worse covers the times of fertility and infertility as well as the times of a sexy-feeling wife and a not-so-sexy wife.

In conclusion, a husband can respond to his wife's changes in sexual desires with understanding, tenderness, affection and appreciation for the mother of his children. He can agree to have sex less and to be more of a helpmate with the baby or to do more activities with the older children. He can also share with his wife in the emotional enjoyment of children by responding to his baby, playing with him, and holding him. She, in turn, can respond with affection and love for her husband, even during lovemaking when her bodily feelings do not seem to be there. I find no reason for extended abstinence simply because the nursing wife does not experience sexual urges. Love is, after all, a decision, not just a feeling.

17

Personal Experiences

There is ample research to show that the breastfeeding program described in these pages will normally be effective in child spacing, but most people are not going to review the sources I have quoted. Most of us learn best by example. Thus I have included the following experiences from friends who initially took an interest in the subject of natural child spacing and who helped me develop my ideas about natural mothering. Although these experiences occurred during the 1960s when the primary emphasis was on child spacing through the "exclusive breastfeeding" rule, their stories show that they were grateful for both the natural infertility and the nursing experience itself.

Their experiences likewise led me to write this book. For some reason, the physicians attending these women could not supply them with the information they needed at the time. They were most grateful for the information they received during our many conversations; and since this information was not available in book form, they encouraged me to put what we talked about into print. The names have been changed.

Ann

Ann completely nursed her baby for five months before gradually introducing solids to her baby. Her first menstrual period occurred when her baby, her fifth, was 14½ months of age.

Ann spotted at about three months postpartum with this baby. And this was repeated 28 days later. Her obstetrician did not believe in the spacing benefit of breastfeeding and told her that her periods were trying to return. She and I were both puzzled by the spotting, as her baby was exclusively breastfed. Finally I asked her when she fed the baby during the night. She replied that her baby went to sleep early in the evening and awoke in the morning, quite content to go without an immediate feeding. We both felt that this long lapse in time may have been the cause of the spotting. She then took my suggestion to nurse her baby before retiring or else first thing in the morning. (I was not encouraging mothers to sleep with their babies at that time. In fact I was totally opposed to anyone sleeping with their baby in those days.) There were nights when her baby was too sleepy to nurse, and then there were nights when he demanded a night feeding. She also tried to increase his daytime feedings. No further signs of spotting or bleeding occurred until 10 months later when she had her first period. Thus she had no menstruation during the months 5 to 14 postpartum while she was giving her baby other foods. Her baby weaned himself at 17 months of age.

Ann could not convince her personal physician of the merit of breastfeeding in the area of family planning. As for her pediatrician, she was very reluctant to tell him that she was still exclusively nursing her baby. At the six-month checkup, she expressed her feelings on the matter and expected that he would advise her to stop nursing. But to her surprise the doctor sat down, asked her questions, and then admitted that he wished all mothers of his little patients would do exactly as she was doing.

The previous babies of Ann and her husband had been born about a year apart. They were happy to learn about natural spacing, for they wanted a larger family at a somewhat slower rate, and both liked the natural way of doing things. It was also this mother who kept insisting that I write a book on the topic; she felt her goal in life at the time was to get other people to do things.

Betty

Betty nursed her baby exclusively for five months. Soon after some solids were introduced, spotting occurred. The mother returned to exclusive breastfeeding and about two months later reintroduced solids because her baby wanted them. A regular period soon followed when her baby was eight months old. This was her fifth baby.

Betty did not believe that breastfeeding would delay the return of fertility. However, after reading the research and realizing that it is the suckling that is so important, she became convinced and was also upset that her doctor hadn't told her about natural spacing with her first baby.

Betty had several comments regarding her early return of menstruation after she introduced solids to her baby. First, she felt that the pacifier was her drawback. Since her baby used the pacifier regularly, he was never content to remain at the breast like other babies. Maybe this additional pacification would have been all that was needed in order to hold back menstruation for a longer period of time after the baby began solids.

Secondly, she often used solids to pacify the baby when all the baby wanted was her. If she was too busy to hold the baby, she found it more convenient to offer food to satisfy him. She came to regard this as a poor form of mothering. It also tended to limit the amount of nursing at the breast by filling up the baby with solids.

Betty found several advantages related to exclusive breastfeeding.

1. She was extremely happy she learned about natural spacing and had peace of mind during the non-menstrual phase of breastfeeding.

2. With her previous babies, she had found carrying them during menstruation very uncomfortable because of leg pains. However, with her last

baby this did not occur due to the absence of menstruation. Also by the time most nursing mothers' periods resume, their babies are learning how to walk and do not need to be carried as much around the house. She felt that other mothers who are uncomfortable during menstruation would also benefit by nursing properly and experiencing a lengthy absence from menstruation.

3. Betty strongly felt that the children are the ones who benefit immensely from the extra contact and attention that is part of natural mothering. She believed it is so much easier to do this when they were little than to try to make up for it in later years. Frequently when babies are born close together, the parents tend to treat the older baby as a grown child and fail to realize that they really have two babies in the house — both needing lots of babying and loving care.

4. And, lastly, she felt that if she had exclusively breastfed in the early months, she would have been able to nurse her other babies. Early introduction of bottles and solids was the cause of her nursing failures. Her 10-month-old looked as if he would be an early weaner; he was nursing well only once during the day. The baby quickly lost interest in the breast once solids were introduced. (Regular use of the pacifier played a part in this also.) Betty planned to nurse until the baby weaned himself; she was enjoying the relationship too much to stop, and she believed that babies should be nursed for about two years. Since in her locality it is extremely rare to hear of a mother still nursing a baby at 10 months of age, she didn't plan to advertise the fact. "I don't feel I have to explain myself to others or want to be in a position where I have to think up some reasons. I just want to and it's as simple as that."

Carol

Carol, a pharmacist from Australia but living in Canada at the time of our meeting, nursed her second child exclusively for seven months. Her periods returned when her baby was nine months old.

Carol absorbed the typical cultural notion that breastfeeding doesn't postpone the return of fertility, so she wanted to quit nursing at three months for fear of becoming pregnant. Thus Carol began to offer her baby some formula. Her female pediatrician asked her why she wanted to stop nursing since her baby was allergic to other milks. She then told Carol about exclusive breastfeeding in order to delay the return of fertility and explained why that would mean delaying solids for some time. She also referred her to me.

As a pharmacist, Carol became extremely interested in the research material on the subject. She then remembered that her grandmother nursed all her children for two to three years and said it was the **only** way, and that her mother's advice was "Be careful when you wean."

It was interesting to note that Carol's baby went an unusually long period of time between feedings for a breastfed baby. Her baby nursed every four to six hours during the day, whereas most babies nurse several times during that amount of time. From five weeks of age her baby slept through the night for 12 to 13 hours. When the baby was four months old, she began to wake him to nurse before she went to bed because she felt that the long time between feedings might force a return of menstruation. However, no bleeding occurred during those early months. (Most mothers would not remain in amenorrhea in a similar situation.)

The attitudes of different doctors who saw this mother were interesting. The pediatrician saw no reason why Carol couldn't exclusively breastfeed her baby for nine months, but her obstetrician thought she was playing "Vatican roulette" and told her she would be lucky if it worked. This doctor regularly told nursing mothers that they should take other precautions or else he would be seeing them next year to deliver another baby. Carol did not convince him, but she relied on breastfeeding in spite of her doctor's opinions and in spite of her not wanting another pregnancy. Finally at her last visit, the obstetrician said that he could see that it might work if a mother had a really aggressive baby — although this mother's baby was certainly not aggressive or very demanding at the breast.

Her general practitioner, on the other hand, was extremely interested in what she had to say and said he really learned something new. This doctor was very happy for her, said he would give the information to other interested patients, and also said he was especially pleased to see a healthy baby who was nursed so long on just mother's milk.

Carol decided to let her baby continue nursing; plans for abrupt weaning gave way to understanding and enjoying the nursing relationship.

Donna

Donna nursed her third baby exclusively for 7½ months. The baby was 11 months old when menstruation returned. She weaned her baby at 16 months of age.

Donna introduced cereal a week before she learned about the spacing benefit of exclusive breastfeeding. She called her pediatrician, and he told her it would be all right to drop the cereal and to exclusively nurse her baby.

In Donna's own words: "Most of all, the child spacing and 100% nursing were the greatest helps." She had nursed her other two babies, but she found that with this baby she had a very different and special relationship due simply to the exclusive breastfeeding. "I think 100% breastfeeding is the only way to start a baby out in this complex world of ours. For me it was the most wonderful experience of motherhood I have ever had."

Author's experience

I wish I could say that someone had given me adequate instruction about breastfeeding with our first child, but the fact is that like most mothers I was really quite ignorant about it. I heard something about exclusive breastfeeding and spacing at La Leche League meetings when I was expecting our first baby, but my obstetrician told me at the time that it didn't work. As a result our first baby was not exclusively breastfed. I used occasional bottles and began solids at five months. She used pacifiers regularly. My first period occurred at three months due to cultural nursing. I thought at the time that this was a natural occurrence because my obstetrician said that no matter how I nursed, I would have a period by three months postpartum. Little did I realize until later how unnatural this early return of menstruation was if you take nature as your norm. Weaning was completed at 10 months of age; in fact during the last two months of nursing I was only able to provide milk at one breast because the use of bottles interfered with lactation. There were times when John encouraged me to nurse instead of relying more and more on the use of bottles.

In those days we were also doing things that are not advocated in this book. John and I were very much a part of our culture. In parenting our first child, we used pacifiers regularly as well as bottles for water and juice. We thought nothing of leaving our first baby in the care of others, and John had somehow gotten the idea that it was beneficial for her to have different sitters. We both felt very strongly that she should have her separate bed and bedroom, and I would never nurse our first baby lying down for fear of smothering her. Nursing at night was a chore since I sat up, often cold and tired. In addition, I was a part-time working mother. Before graduation (1962) at a major state university and medical center, my classmates and I were told by our professional staff at an evening meeting that we dental hygienists should continue to work when we had children, that we owed it to society since the state had put so much money into our education.

I had planned on permanently leaving my job after the birth of our first child, but one of my bosses made a special plea for my return, and I resumed work two afternoons a week. Even then, however, I could never understand how my classmates could leave their babies all day. One friend worked for her orthodontist-husband full days, and I remember trying to convince her to work only half-days because of her baby. A half-day was long enough for me, and if history could repeat itself, I would stay at home where I belonged. John and I have changed considerably in our growth as parents.

We did have a two-year spacing between our first two children, but that was due to two miscarriages in between. One of the miscarriages occurred when I was nursing. I wondered if the nursing caused the miscarriage, but I was informed by the local medical doctors I spoke with and also by La Leche League International that nursing is not a factor in a miscarriage.

After our second baby was born, I picked up considerably more information about exclusive breastfeeding. As a result, I exclusively nursed for the first time. I also started sleeping with our baby for naps and night nursings, a practice I would not consider with our first child. This baby did not use a pacifier. My periods started at 12 months postpartum. While nursing this baby, I was also encouraged by the fact that I knew two other mothers who exclusively nursed their babies while I was doing so. One of the mothers was Ann mentioned previously; the other mother nursed exclusively for nine months and her menstruation returned at 18 months. She was still nursing and giving night feedings at this age. Menstruation for all three of us did not resume until our babies were 12 to 18 months old.

My new obstetrician with our second baby advocated exclusive breast-feeding to avoid a pregnancy only because he knew I wanted to nurse this baby. He merely said: "Give her nothing but your milk, not even water." And he added: "Call me when you have your first period." I never did call him a year later because we were in the process of moving and we were once again thinking of another baby.

When I informed our pediatrician of my plans for our second baby, he was most interested, since he admitted not knowing anything about it. During our visits he never once made a reference to solids or juices. When the baby rejected the vitamin drops, he said that they were not that important but that I should make sure my diet was good. He admitted not having learned anything about breastfeeding in his training, but was most impressed by the breastfed babies in his practice. He checked her iron after she reached six months of age and found everything satisfactory. Most of all, he was pleased with her overall health and good disposition.

I admired this particular doctor — not only for his interest in breast-feeding — but for a special reason: he respected my right to decide when I should offer my baby something besides breastmilk. I hinted, and even asked for his opinion as to when I should begin solids. He never answered that question. Neither he nor my husband would offer an opinion, other than letting me know I was free to go as long as I desired and as long as the baby continued to thrive on breastmilk. The decision was entirely mine. At eight months, our baby showed her first tooth, so I took this eruption to mean a time for weaning. At least it became the answer to my question, 'How long?' However, if the tooth had erupted at four or six months of age, I would have ignored this sign. If the baby were unhappy and needed the solids, I would have begun solids earlier. The introduction of solids at such a late date in no way detracted from her health or disposition. Only her mother knew when people commented how well she must eat or asked if she was that good all the time.

Our girl thus became familiar with non-milk foods and took a sip occasionally from a cup. I continued to offer the breast so that she was still receiving most of her liquid diet from me. At age 18 months she came down with a cold, and I took advantage of the opportunity to wean her. That type of forced weaning is inconsistent with what I recommend in this book, and I have done it differently with our last three children.

Our third baby was born when our second was 24 months old. She was also nursed exclusively for eight months, at which time she began to take some solids. Menstruation returned at 10½ months — exactly 14 days after she had a large decrease in appetite for any food including breastmilk. This reduction in the amount of suckling for a two-day period caused, I believe, a premature return of menstruation. At about this time we came across a natural family planning article by Dr. Konald A. Prem from the University of

Minnesota Medical School. Little did we know then that this doctor later would be instrumental in helping us start the Couple to Couple League so we could share information about natural family planning and ecological breastfeeding with other couples.

Our fourth and fifth children, like our third child, were nursed exclusively for eight months and I followed the ecological breastfeeding program described in this book. I am convinced from my reading of the literature and from our parenting experiences that natural mothering via breastfeeding provides the best start for the baby as well as the mother and that breastfeeding almost always provides a rich emotional development for both mother and baby. The frequent and unrestricted nursing associated with natural mothering usually provides a natural spacing of births of about two to three years.

The need for the seven standards

You will notice that the emphasis in these personal accounts from the mid-to-late 60s are primarily on exclusive breastfeeding. Then "exclusive breastfeeding" was the only rule given if you wanted to delay fertility. These accounts were from friends who were learning about exclusive breastfeeding and applying it in their personal lives. However, I would like to stress, as I have said previously, that exclusive breastfeeding during the first six months of life is only one piece of the "natural infertility pie." While this aspect of breastfeeding is important, the other six standards advocated in this book are of equal importance in maintaining postpartum infertility.

In my discussions with other interested mothers, it soon became apparent that other factors contributed to child spacing since many mothers in a bottlefeeding culture have a return of their periods while exclusively breastfeeding. During the parenting of our second and third children, we discovered many of the natural mothering concepts and gradually developed the ecological breastfeeding program. In the late sixties and early seventies, "ecology" was almost like a new religion; it was constantly in the news media with regard to pollution and population. It seemed appropriate at that time to coin the term "ecological breastfeeding" to stress nature's way and to set it apart from the cultural nursing of most American mothers. Thus the exclusive breastfeeding rule eventually became just one of the Seven Standards of the ecological breastfeeding program.

The Mailbox

Mothers who have written me after reading this book have three themes running through their letters: 1) they lack support from doctors and relatives; 2) they are deeply appreciative for the information and support given by the Couple to Couple League and its magazine, *CCL Family Foundations*, and by La Leche League, and 3) they experienced longer amenorrhea by following the natural plan for mothering. Here are some excerpts from letters written by mothers mostly from the United States but also from Canada, Australia, and New Zealand. The quotes are essentially unedited. I share these letters because I think that these experiences and thoughts offer support to mothers involved with ecological breastfeeding. They make the principles come alive.

Natural child spacing

"God didn't mean for women to become baby-factories, giving birth to a new child every year. In order that our bodies could recuperate from childbirth and build up strength for a next pregnancy, He planned that breastfeeding would render us infertile for one to two years. Why should we bother with foams, artificial devices or the pill? God's plan is so much nicer!"

"You may also wonder if I am of a faith that does not condone birth control means. No, I am not, and I have in fact taken the pill for a year and a half between my two children. My boys are over three years apart, as I remained sterile for nearly a year after those pills. So I've found breastfeeding a lovely blessing in every way, and the infertility is only a convenient side effect. We've decided on a third child at the earliest possible date — considering the breastfeeding situation, of course."

"I want to thank you for writing the book *Breastfeeding and Natural Child Spacing*. What a Godsend! My youngest is almost 18 months old now, and I still have not experienced my first postpartum period! I only wish I had known of this with my other children."

"I'd just like to say I feel certain breastfeeding has a very definite effect on child spacing. With my bottlefed children I conceived again at eight months after delivery despite other contraceptives. So far it has been 15 months since the last baby was born. No period yet."

"I first read your book when Lynda had nearly weaned herself. It certainly makes sense, and I am looking forward to having another baby. I only wish I had known more when Lynda was a baby because contraception can be such a worry. I would never go on the pill again."

"My husband and I are very pleased with this most natural means of spacing children. It is especially great these hectic months after birth when tension over effectiveness of other methods and adjustments to a new baby can put a strain on a marriage. We feel this way is best for our family in every way and are overjoyed it works so well."

"Our 15-month-old is still nursing three or four times a day. For a while it seemed he wasn't too interested, except early in the morning. I haven't had a period yet. The other day someone was complaining of cramps and discomfort with her period, and I mentioned that since my first baby I have never had all that cramping and pain with my periods. Then I said, 'But come to think of it, I've had so few periods.' And my friend said, 'You know, you are the truly liberated woman!' How true! So far I have had 11 periods in over eight years. That is with three babies."

"I just finished reading your book. Very informative! I just wish I could have read it 20 years ago! Our little girl wakes at night to be nursed and sometimes nurses often at night. We have a king-size bed so it really doesn't bother our sleep. We have relied entirely on nursing for postponing pregnancy. It is the most enjoyable method of spacing babies. I just regret all the years that were completely safe or could have been and we didn't know it."

"As a Protestant, it had never been presented to my husband and me as a logical way to have a family. Our sweet little one is nine days old, and she will be the first one not to have a soother [pacifier]. Many of my acquaintances are put right on the IUD after their first baby, and I think it's a shame when God intended His way of spacing little ones."

"This is the only method of child spacing that appeals to my husband and me in every possible way. Myself, I look for simpler answers — ones that women in nontechnological societies might discover — and in breastfeeding I found it."

"Perhaps the future of the family is at stake in this generation, but I have faith in God that perhaps some of the turmoil the world is going through will make us return to the warmth and love, the heartaches and the pride that can come only from close family unity. Developing as human beings is the only thing that can have meaning in a world that so often labels us as numbers. Breastfeeding and natural family planning can give us direction as families by turning us toward humanness."

"Nursing Lisa has been a beautiful experience. She is a wonderful, contented baby. Her weight gain has been well above normal and her iron level measured at six months was fine. She gave up that 2:00 a.m. feed very early at about six weeks. At three months she gave up the 10:00 p.m. feed, so I had that long stretch without nursing at night again. I went back to night feedings but she gave up one of her daytime feedings so I was still on four feeds a day. I spasmodically fed her at night but it was obvious she did not want it. I finally gave up and she seemed happier. At six months she went to three feeds a day with four every now and then. I began solids around 5½ months with small pieces of banana and gradually introduced other foods. Lisa was ready for solids and took to them greedily. I always nursed her before solids. Now she eats three meals a day and I cut out her midday nursing. However, she has been sick, and the last three nights with high fever she has gone back to nursing as nothing else makes her happy. One would expect a return of periods and/or ovulation with such a decrease in nursing, but apparently I must be able to keep the levels of inhibitory hormone high enough to prevent ovulation."

"My second child is now 7½ months old. I haven't had a period yet. I exclusively breastfed him until 6½ months when he wanted food from my plate. I learned from experience that I must be careful about solids. My baby nurses twice at night and for long periods of time."

"Our fourth baby was born at home because we wanted no interference with hospital schedules. Because of this we nursed almost continually from a few minutes after birth until she was 25 hours old. The only times she wasn't at breast were when I was otherwise occupied — i.e., changing pads. This was beautiful for both of us. My milk was in at 16 hours and she passed all the black stool by two days of age. She (6½ months old) is now having one meal of solids per day. This is mainly meat, a few ounces of our regular table food. She has never slept in a bed other than ours since birth. She nurses on and off during the night, but I really don't know how often. I sleep nude from the waist up, so does the baby, in order to allow more skin contact. Consequently she nurses whenever she likes. We use no other form of birth control so I imagine our next baby will come along in two years. My husband and I are both enjoying this fourth baby. It's my husband's idea to have her sleep with us. He feels she will benefit greatly by the close cuddling she gets at night. With three other children to care for, he feels the baby may not get enough holding and loving during the day. Therefore, he wants to ensure her getting her share of me at night."

"It has been my observation in three years of talking to nursing mothers, that night feedings are a critical factor in extending the time of postpartum amenorrhea, and that taking the baby to bed with you is a critical factor in extending night feedings. May I make a suggestion? It helps to stop thinking in terms of the bedroom and consider a sleeping room, with safe, low mattresses where the baby always sleeps. Then supplement this with a nearby, comfortable area to which the husband and wife may retire if they wish privacy. Many of the overwhelming problems of breastfeeding are really problems of logistics — confining floor plans, furniture, and clothes which dictate a lifestyle that conflicts with breastfeeding."

"This was the first baby exclusively breastfed for six months, and also a true baby-led weaning. The assurance I got from my husband was what I needed. He really acted as a buffer against the relatives and friends. My doctor was a tremendous help by his positive attitude. It also helped to be able to quote his remarks to the relatives. The baby nursed very infrequently, but gained three pounds every month for the first six months except one month he gained four pounds. I am currently nursing our 17-month-old without a return of my periods."

"I believe not only in lying down while nursing but also in sleeping with one's children. My son nursed on and off during the nights. He is 22 months old and I have not yet had a period. Sleeping with one's children is so easy, so natural, so safe, and so warm and loving."

"We are not new to CCL. In fact, we have been using ecological mothering and natural child spacing since January of 1988 when our second child was born. We have relied solely on natural child spacing since then. Our youngest was conceived after we sought advice from CCL following two miscarriages back to back. After the two miscarriages we doubted we would ever have another child. That child did become a reality. Since her birth we have again been engaged in ecological mothering enjoying not only the natural infertility as planned by God but also the wonderful closeness and bonding that can only be achieved by such a relationship."

"I have yet to finish your book, but I am now following your instructions for ecological breastfeeding to a 'T'. I sleep with my daughter, nurse her at least two times a night and often during the day. I have rarely left her side since she was born. I even shower with her, using a shower sling, and I use a carrier often. My daughter was very cranky and cried a lot about three weeks ago. The security of being held in my arms or in the carrier or by my husband, I believe, 'cured' the problem. *(continued)*

I love your coverage of real, natural mothering. People tell me I hold my baby too much, feed her too often, should give her a pacifier, should not sleep with her, etc. I ignore it all. How can my family possibly be happier?

My religion, Islam, encourages breastfeeding for two years and, according to some Muslim scholars, allows birth control to be practiced within that two-year period. I feel that so many people ignore breastfeeding as a form of natural child spacing. The techniques you describe are entirely compatible with my religion."

"Here is a check for more charts. Everything has been going so well! I just had my first postpartum cycle following the birth of my almost-18-month-old son. Everything clicked right back on. After both children, I had no transition period. Just a few weeks of unmistakable mucus to get my attention, then right back to normal cycles. I was very pleased. After such a long time without charting (26 months), I was afraid a transitory time would really challenge my skills. I've only had 10 periods in 6½ years. Our daughter is 4½. We used the method for over two years before we conceived her, so it's definitely worked well for us. We are not Catholic."

"My daughter, our first child, was nursed for 14 months. She called a nursing strike and I was unsuccessful in getting her to nurse again. She's very strong-willed. I resumed menstruation at 15 months and then conceived my son who at 22 months is still an avid nurser. I have yet to have a postpartum menstrual cycle since his birth. I'm in no hurry to wean him. We are relying on breastfeeding alone as our method of child spacing."

"In Tahiti breastfeeding was practically extinct, so we were an oddity. The available juice had sugar so I didn't want my son drinking it. The cow's milk was unsafe and the water was dirty. That left breastmilk which was safe and available. Now at age 3½, he is bright, healthy, and very secure. I never left him until he said he was ready for me to go which was at age 2½, and then I only left him with familiar family members. I now have a second son, and again we use only breastfeeding for birth spacing and my period has not returned."

"My daughter is 13 months old and we're enjoying the breastfeeding relationship. I like the amenorrhea, and my husband and I are pleased with the absence of artificial birth control. I am enjoying full-time mothering following four years as a social worker. My husband is a new family practice physician. He promotes breastfeeding at every opportunity and out of personal conviction does not prescribe the Pill or fit IUDs for patients.

I have not always found support for natural mothering among fellow Christians nor have I found much overt support for Christianity in the literature on breastfeeding and natural mothering. Your book helped to cement my conviction that this way is truly God's intended way of parenting.

153

[Childcare] is just one more area where the world has influenced the Church rather than the other way around. As for being pro-life and a 'natural' mother, I believe it's the only consistent line of thought and behavior based on love for children."

"My 14½ month old daughter and I are still enjoying our nursing relationship, and although my doctor assured me I was normal, I was concerned about my continued infertility. Many people had said, 'Don't count on it for birth control,' so I didn't. As it turned out, I can! I picked up your book out of curiosity and to better understand what my body was experiencing. I am very reassured to know that rather than being unusual, breastfeeding infertility is natural, normal and healthy. Why don't doctors know this stuff? Why did my obstetrician, who encouraged breastfeeding, ask me at six weeks postpartum if I'd like to wean and go on the Pill? Life is full of questions, isn't it!"

"Although I am a registered nurse who graduated three years ago, I was not taught about the relationship between breastfeeding and lactation amenorrhea. In fact, I remember being taught to tell new mothers that 'Breastfeeding is not a reliable way to prevent pregnancy and to use contraception.' I feel very angry about this now. How unfair to people who would be interested in spacing their children naturally if the information were made available to them! How can we get the nursing and medical schools to teach their students the facts about natural child spacing through breastfeeding and to take natural family planning seriously?"

"I want to thank you for responding so promptly to my letter seeking advice on weaning my then 26-month-old son. As you suggested, I got back in touch with a nearby La Leche League and at one of the meetings I received some helpful advice. I appreciated your encouragement to continue following child-led weaning. I had a period a couple of days after writing to you. It was the first one following 26 months of amenorrhea. I was ecstatic, almost as excited as I was at age 14 when I had my first menstrual period! I began charting immediately, ovulated and conceived soon after. I did wean our son during my pregnancy, but at a pace that suited us both. I thought when our daughter arrived he would desire to nurse but he hasn't seemed to. He snuggles with us as we nurse and instructs me to nurse when she has the hiccups or cries. I do hope he will be a supportive husband to a breastfeeding wife and mom one day."

Mother-baby togetherness
"My baby sucked her fingers a lot the first three months when I tried halfheartedly to follow a schedule. She stopped when I really relaxed and nursed her as often and as long as she needed."

"Last summer when I was seven months pregnant, my father died suddenly of a heart attack, leaving me to run the family retail business with my younger brother. I decided I had to carry on the business he had worked so hard to establish. I was determined to take the baby to work with me. He slept contentedly most of the time, and when he needed to nurse, I took him into an adjoining room where we had privacy. As time went on, people began to remark on how placid and friendly he was. As for me, I never felt or looked better in my life. I was bursting with energy. So much for all the stories that breastfeeding is tiring and takes so much out of you."

"Here on the Air Force base, when a woman is pregnant, one of her priorities is finding a babysitter. We are considered strange because our baby is always with us. Our most difficult situations have been military functions. We carry the baby and ignore the odd glances. We like to make our ideas known in a gentle way when talking to people, but are careful not to be pushy or obnoxious. We have attended two formal military functions with the baby. In those cases we brought along a young 12-year-old friend who cared for him in the lobby of the officers' club. I slipped away from time to time. We have found that our style of parenting requires more creativity, but obstacles can usually be overcome. Sometimes an activity must be given up temporarily."

"I have five breastfed children, but it wasn't always easy. With the first one I felt very tied down with breastfeeding. I made sure she would take a bottle so I could get out and get away once in a while. When I look back now, the problem was that I wasn't comfortable nursing around others. I have overcome this. I have taken my nursing babies to concerts and picnics — even to the Democratic County Convention. Going on nature hikes is easy with a nursing baby. I've nursed the baby at church by covering the baby with a blanket.

Our last three babies slept with us for two years. Even though I'm 38 now and have a five-month-old, I've never felt tired like I did with our first one who slept in a crib in a separate room. It's also nice to nurse the baby and read to a preschooler at the same time. The truth has set me free."

"I must admit there are some things I will not do again. First, I will never leave my baby with a sitter. I was pressured by our society rather than following my own instinct here. I also really resisted sleeping with my baby. But because of my illness and the baby's illness, we came to family sleeping and I discovered how wonderful it could be! I certainly got more sleep, and she seemed to sleep better with us than in her own room."

"I believe our daughter is above average in intelligence. I realize I may not be objective, but I hear the same thing from many other people who have come in contact with her. She is very friendly and outgoing and likes to play with other children or adults. This is in spite of (I believe because of) my staying home with her and never leaving her with sitters to get away. She's been going with me to football and basketball games since she was three weeks old while other parents leave their kids with a sitter."

"Joshua has been a real joy. He's been to the mountains, the Gulf of Mexico, flown in an airplane, and helped me drive the combine at age six weeks. Truly a portable, happy, easy-to-care-for baby. I'll never go back to cribs and bottles."

"In 1980 my husband and I went to Italy and France with our four-year-old daughter and nine-month-old son. Many tour groups do not allow young children on their tours, so we did a lot of research about where we wanted to go and what we wanted to do and went on our own. We had planned this trip as far back as when I was pregnant with Paul. When our plan to travel became known to friends and family, it was met with mixed reactions. Some thought it was a neat idea to take our kids, and some thought we were crazy. We didn't think it would be a burden since I nursed Paul.

Since we had plenty of time to plan, we figured out how many disposable diapers to take, how much clothing would be needed, and what we would carry around on a daily basis in a backpack. We purchased a Gerry carrier so I could comfortably carry Paul and still have my hands free. The airlines arranged for us to have a 'sky cradle' so Paul could have a place to sleep during our transatlantic flight.

We had a wonderful time and having the children along proved to be a real blessing. Everywhere we went, the people went out of their way to make sure we had what we needed and that we got good seats on the trains and local transportation. Everyone stopped to smile at our family, to hug the kids, and to make conversation. Whenever necessary, I was able to nurse Paul, and I never had to worry about formulas or local food that might make him sick. It really was no problem for us. Nursing Paul provided an easy way for us to travel. All it took was planning and organization to make a successful trip.

Now we have three children (ages 8, 4, and 2) and we are planning to go to Italy this summer. Even though I won't be nursing a child on this trip, it is nice to know if I were, it would not keep me from traveling."

"First I want to thank you for the positive effect you've had on my mothering skills. I nursed my first baby for 4½ months and then quit because of the inconvenience. I nursed my second baby for 22 months because it was so very convenient. The only thing that changed was my attitude and finding a supportive group of friends.

When our second baby was seven or eight months old, we had our annual family reunion at a campground. My two sisters had babies one month younger than mine and watching them at this camp-out made me thankful I was nursing. They were constantly warming up bottles by heating water on the Coleman stove (no fast procedure) and worrying about saving opened bottles in the ice chest and wondering how long they would keep safely. Then once a day my two sisters worked together washing and sterilizing bottles and nipples, and again needed to heat water on the Coleman stove. At night one sister warmed a bottle and put it under her sweatshirt so she could keep it warm for her baby's night feeding. She didn't want to heat a bottle at 1:00 a.m. I won't mention the process involved in fixing their cereals and baby food, but it too was time consuming.

Compare their methods of feeding to my method which was breast-feeding. All I needed to do when my baby was hungry was to find a place to sit. Night feedings were even easier. My husband and I zipped our two sleeping bags together and there was room for the three of us. When the baby whimpered, he was immediately satisfied and we were both back to sleep within minutes.

When our second child was a year old, we drove 10 hours from Michigan to Iowa. I could nurse him without unbuckling his car seat. I'd have to take my seat belt off though. Again nursing was very convenient. We usually would stop the car to nurse because it was more comfortable for me to hold him in my arms. And our three year old appreciated the nursing breaks as he got to get out of the car and play with dad. Also my periods resumed at 20 months postpartum. I enjoyed not having periods for that long."

"My insistence on staying with my 10-month-old daughter landed us an unplanned appearance in Paramount Pictures' *The Hunter*, which was Steve McQueen's last film! It was filmed in the Chicago area in the fall of 1980. Some of my family members are models and had landed parts as extras for the three weeks of filming in Chicago. After the Chicago filming, the set moved to some rural areas near Kankakee, where we lived. When my mom (who was in the filming) heard that they were coming down, she suggested that they call me to help find people for the stand-in parts.

The agent asked me to come and take a part. 'No,' I said, 'I have a 10-month-old nursing baby.' 'It's only for a half day,' he responded. I knew this meant seven or eight hours to them. 'That's too long to leave her,' I said as my heart sank. He told me it would be O.K. to come and watch, and bring her if she's quiet.

As we observed the filming at the Kankakee Airport, the assistant director got an idea. Although he did not know me at all, he picked my baby and me from the observing crowd and told us to be in the next scene. We rehearsed a few times and discovered we would be in a scene with Steve McQueen. There were four of us and the pilot in the small plane. I sat across from Steve McQueen, knee-to-knee, with Susie on my lap. He mentioned how good she was and talked about his own daughter. Throughout the rehearsals, the shuttles, the practicing getting off and back on the plane, and being passed around, Susie was an angel.

Knowing that many hours of taped scenes are always cut from the final film, I was surprised to see Susie and myself in the premiere showing ten months later. A still shot of our scene with McQueen holding Susie returns again at the very last background for the credits at the end of the film.

Of all the stand-ins available, our mother-baby togetherness was the key to this once-in-a-lifetime experience for us. A few months after the filming, we received in the mail a large laminated wall plaque with a photo of our scene. It is personally inscribed 'To Colleen and Susie, from a fan... Steve McQueen.' The following October, McQueen died of cancer. It was truly a privilege to have met this man and experienced some of his kindness toward children."

"I have followed mother-baby closeness with both Owen and Paul, and I believe that it was a big help to their development and to their sense of security. I can see my children developing into loving people who value people over things — that is the way we have treated them. It seems to me that those parents who reject natural mothering may be saying that there is only so much giving that can be expected and 'I have my own life to live. This baby isn't going to change everything about my life!' Although this seems very selfish to me, many mothers feel entirely justified in this belief.

Then there are those mothers who believe the best thing for their babies is to be taught to be a 'good baby' whereas I believe my babies will teach me to be a good mother. I think these mothers are sincere in trying to do what is best, although from my perspective that seems to be what is most convenient. Eventually the baby will sleep through the night and will be comfortable with lengthening separations from mom.

If we are called to see Christ in everyone, then we should certainly see the baby Jesus in our babies. I often ask myself how would the Blessed Mother handle this or that problem. Thanks for bringing this part of natural family planning to so many mothers."

"My husband and I had it all planned. We would have a baby in a hospital and I would nurse for several months. The baby would sleep all night by three months of age and we would have a regular sitter so we could go out. Little did we know how parenthood would change us. We listened to each other and grew. Decisions were often painful and difficult to make.

Adam was born to us in an alternative birthing center. The three of us were never separated, and we returned home the same day he was born. We needed our baby near us and we often brought him to bed with us for those night nursings. At age two weeks he developed colic and the family bed became reality as a matter of survival.

Adam did not do well without me. He needed me intensely and I was unable to leave him even for an hour. He nursed about every 1½ to 2 hours around the clock for 10 months. I knew from my LLL group that I was

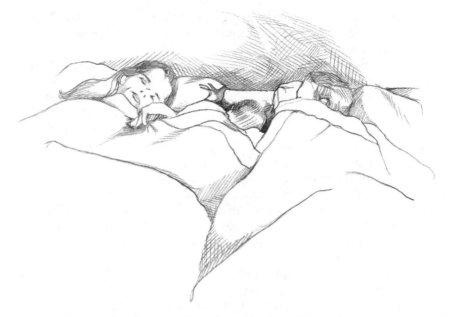

meeting the needs of my child and yet I often felt inadequate. It seemed other mothers had extra time for showers, reading and cooking. Adam's naps were often only 20 minutes long. This led to many feelings of frustration and anger. And yet, as we watched Adam grow, we knew we were making right decisions even though our family and friends often disagreed with us.

Adam went everywhere with us. He attended weddings, parties, meetings, and peace rallies. Now at 15 months he is very active, happy and friendly. He still goes almost everywhere with us, but once in a while we leave him with friends for a couple of hours to take in a movie. He seems secure with this and does just fine. As for natural mothering, we would do it all over again. It does take support of like-minded friends and a dedicated spirit."

"First, I'd like to give you an idea of my background. I worked in a technical career involving computers and mathematics for about seven years prior to the birth of my first child two years ago. I was convinced of the importance of a child being raised at home by a parent, yet I had a strong need to maintain my career and stay technically oriented. I decided to fulfill both needs by staying home with my daughter during the day and getting my doctorate on a part-time basis (two evenings a week) while my husband watched the baby. Clare was never without one parent until we went out to dinner when she was seven months old and we left her with a sitter.

From 7 to 17 months, she was left with a sitter no more than three or four times. I decided to attend a technical seminar for three days when Clare was 17 months old. This meant I was away from her from 7 to 9 hours per day. I wasn't that worried about leaving her since my parents were coming down to watch her and she was able to go that long without nursing. It was while I attended this seminar that I found out the primary benefit of mother-baby togetherness.

The first morning of the seminar I nursed Clare in bed as usual. After she finished she did her typical hugging and caressing me. All I could think of was how hard it would be to leave her. Clare got along great with my parents and I had an enjoyable time at the seminar, so much so that visions of going back to work full-time danced in my head. However, what really made me reconsider was how Clare treated me after the seminar was over. She still nursed as often as usual, but the hugging and caressing had stopped. Not only that but at times she even preferred to play with my mother rather than with me. I thought what it would be like to have Clare be more responsive to a total stranger (i.e., a babysitter I'd have hired) rather than her own mother. Fortunately, the three-day seminar did not totally shatter our relationship. After spending an entire day with Clare, the loving relationship continued where it left off.

I enjoy being at home and watching my child grow both physically and mentally before my eyes. I feel more in tune with my child's needs and can raise her the way I want instead of being at the mercy of her caretaker. I'm not worried about her safety or possible abuse because she is always with us or is cared for occasionally by a person whom we trust.

The most difficult aspect of mother-baby togetherness involves taking our baby along to some events at which she is not really welcome. It's hard to find friends who share the same values that you do. The first few times I left Clare with her father or sitter proved to be pretty traumatic for her and me alike. I don't know who missed whom more. Even now I have a tendency to put off getting a sitter for a night out because there is still some separation anxiety for both of us.

Sometimes I wonder whether we're doing the right things for our daughter. She tends to be shyer than other children who are with others on a regular basis. Having to cope with criticism from the grandparents who feel our daughter should be weaned or that we pay too much attention to her makes things difficult on occasion. Fortunately, the Couple to Couple League conference in Baltimore helped reinforce that we are doing the best possible thing for our daughter."

"We have one daughter who is 2½ years old and who is still nursing. She has gone everywhere with us since she's been born and really it has been no problem. In fact we are so at ease knowing that she is with us and having her needs met by us that the word babysitter is an obsolete word in our household.

The first public place we took Mary was to church. At first I was not comfortable nursing in public so I asked our priests to please put a chair in the church's bathroom. I asked them if they thought they would enjoy nursing a baby on a toilet seat. They gladly obliged. Later as I became more relaxed and more adept at discreetly nursing, I stayed in church and nursed.

Other outings included eating at restaurants. We would bring Mary along and set her in her infant seat. If she needed to be fed, I simply put a receiving blanket over my shoulder and proceeded to nurse her. I do remember the first time I nursed her at a restaurant. I was not real good at getting her started while being discreet about it at the same time. I simply excused myself, took her to the restroom and got her started there. Once she was on, I returned to the table and we both enjoyed our meals. That is a great advantage of breastfeeding — you have one hand free to feed yourself if your little one is also hungry at your mealtime.

Once when we were at a restaurant I noticed another mother nursing her baby. She had situated herself in an out of the way corner of the restaurant. She had a much more comfortable spot to nurse in than I did. Our table was out in the middle of the floor. I felt very conspicuous. That situation taught me a lesson. In the future when we dined out, my husband always asked the hostess to put us in a corner or at least along a wall if possible.

My husband, Mary and I have also gone together to see movies at our local theater. We go to the 9:15 p.m. show. That way we know she will be tired and ready to nurse herself to sleep.

Ours is a large family so we have had the opportunity to take Mary to several weddings and wedding receptions. During the church service we usually sit towards the rear so an exit is easy if necessary. This is very important now that she has entered the trying-two age. Oftentimes church services are very difficult because they don't offer too much excitement for a two year old. We simply recognize this fact and remain flexible. At the reception we come prepared with an appropriate size chair for her to sit in and her own spoon and fork. She has always loved all the excitement that goes along with wedding receptions. When it is obvious that she is tired, we either leave or put her in her portable buggy. Even with all the noise going on around her, she has never had any problem falling asleep.

As you can see, we have fun taking Mary along with us. All that is necessary is a little advance planning so that we bring everything along that will make our outing comfortable for her."

"Jennifer went everywhere with us. The fact that I had to work part-time as a secretary-bookkeeper for the school district did not hamper my mothering style. Through the suggestions of the district administrator, we worked out a unique working relationship. Our baby was a 'colicky' baby; she nursed frequently and suckled endlessly. My husband's union contract was ending with talks of a strike, so I knew I had to keep working. While I was on my postnatal leave, the administrator brought my work to my home. I stretched my vacation days to reduce my workdays. When that ended, Jenny was still colicky and I was frazzled by the rush-rush pace. My boss then suggested coming in on Saturdays with baby, and my husband could care for her while I worked. *(continued)*

So Saturday was an excursion to school. We made ourselves at home in the administrator's office and between feedings I did the district's bookkeeping. Jenny had many hours of backpacking and crawling tours of the school classrooms. She was rocked to sleep in the Executive chair. The Home Ec. room was our kitchen for lunch. An impossible situation to combine work with mothering was solved for a short duration. It was the first in this school district. I am most thankful to the administrator and his suggestion to bring the baby!"

"Emily would not take a pacifier or any bottle. She would only nurse. Therefore, she went everywhere with us. This was fine with my husband and me, and our baby was happy and content. When she was three months old, we had a chance to go to Puerto Rico. Children were not allowed on the trip, but we were going to try to take Emily anyway. When we arrived at the hotel, the man in charge of all the arrangements asked me if I had received the letter explaining 'no children.' I told him our baby came with us because she was exclusively breastfed. He seemed to be concerned about all the 'needs' the baby would need. I said we do not need a baby bed, food, or sterilized bottles. We were not allowed in the casinos nor allowed to see a stage show because no children were allowed. One evening when everyone else went to a show, we were given our dinner 'on the house.' The room was private with candlelight. We had two guests: a little girl and her babysitter. The little girl belonged to the man in charge! He had brought his own daughter along on the trip.

Another time we took her on a couples' retreat for the weekend. She slept with us and never cried during the night because of the nursing. I felt good about taking her because her needs were being met."

"Our biggest challenge was the acceptance from others of our baby being with us. A cross-country ski group attracted us because of their encouragement of family activities. At three months of age Dusty went to Cragun's in Brainerd, Minnesota for a skiing escapade. Many club members remarked on how good he was for the six-hour bus trip there, the skiing itself, and the return bus trip. It is not hard when kids learn to be with mom and dad in all their activities. Just last week, we again trekked to Brainerd. This time Dusty was on skis and his eight-month-old sister was in a Gerry carrier on our backs. We had a great time and enjoyed the family experience. We had bicycled across the United States in 1978, but we are now considering doing it again with the children."

"We have raised our baby the 'hard way' — no baby swings, no pacifiers, and seldom am I out of her sight. Everyone tells me how carefree and easy those babyswings are and say that I am making life harder without one. I don't tell them it frightens me to see their baby with a trancelike stare on its face—back and forth, back and forth for an hour! Yikes."

"Monica has ridden in my back pack as I picked vegetables, canned and froze them. She sits in the flour and squeals at her 'white cloud' as I make bread. I still laugh when I think of her at nine months on my hip as I mashed strawberries in a large bowl. She tried and tried and stretched and tried some more to put her toes in my strawberries!

My husband and I both enjoy the simple things of life. I am happy to afford the luxury of staying home to raise my family. My husband's income is nothing extravagant, but then popcorn, pork and beans, and garden vegetables are good enough for the three of us."

"When I was Director of Pregnancy Aid of Washington State and the WIC program for several counties, I realized how difficult it was for many of the women who were working with me to leave their children in daycare. By then all of my children were in school. I established the policy at all Pregnancy Aid offices for both paid and volunteer staff that children could accompany mothers to work. The only stipulation was that the work get done and that the mother make certain the child did not interfere with the work of others.

When our sixth child was born, I took him to work with me from the time he was three weeks old. There were a few raised eyebrows when it was necessary for me to attend meetings at the State Health Department and when I sat breastfeeding, but the program was efficiently and effectively run, and people adapted very quickly. It makes much more sense to me to see those who are involved in the work force adapt to the needs of children than vice versa.

When our seventh child was born, we flew out with the baby for a job interview. We were asked what we would do with our younger children if we were to assume the position. We explained very clearly and carefully that they would, of course, go to work with us. It made no sense to us to be directing programs devoted to the enrichment of marriage and family and to put our children in daycare.

Shortly after taking the job, we found that some people had either not heard or not assumed that we were serious in bringing our children to work, and there was a bit of a question as to whether this would be allowed to continue. We again made it very clear that our children would come to work with us if we were going to work there.

That was two years ago. Our two boys still play (usually quietly) in the corner of our office. There are still some raised eyebrows. After all, a two year old and a four year old carrying their lunch pails to work down the corridors of a university is not yet considered usual practice.

I do believe, however, that most parents could take their children to work with them. I have talked with a number of people in the last few years who have seen this practice increasing. One woman has said that in her doctor's office, the nurse brings her infant child to work. Others have mentioned other offices where this is becoming the practice. I realize this is not

163

standard, but I do feel that at every opportunity it should be promoted and that it could become eventually the norm rather than the exception."

"When Molly was 11 months old I received a call from my mother asking me if I would like to accompany her, my father, brother, and sister on a pilgrimage to Mexico City to the Shrine of Our Lady of Guadalupe. There was one stipulation: I would have to wean Molly. My mother did not feel it would work out as far as safety, hotel, and traveling if I were to bring her along. I gave it much thought and decided that if I could not take Molly along, I would not go. Our nursing relationship meant too much to me. When my mother saw how determined I was and how much it meant to me, she agreed that I could bring the baby.

We flew to Mexico City while Molly nursed and slept the whole time. Molly and I shared a room with my sister at the hotel. I never had to worry about what she ate or what she drank. She never got sick as many tourists do from the food and water. I carried her in a cloth baby carrier as we toured the city. She was as good as gold; the people there stopped me on the streets to look at her. If I got tired, there were plenty of willing family members to help out. We visited the Shrine, the Pyramids, and several sites throughout the city. We had such a good time."

"When Sarah was only one month old, my husband and I were asked to give talks at the pre-marriage weekends that are held in our town. Since the schedule involved two fairly long days away from home, I could see no possible way of doing the weekends and still be the kind of mother I wished to be. My husband and I felt that we were called to share our marriage with engaged couples, so after a lot of praying we found a solution. We hired a babysitter and took Sarah with us. Our babysitter took care of Sarah while we gave the talks. I was able to nurse her and hold her during breaks and other talks. An additional benefit that I hadn't realized was the engaged couples were able to see another important aspect of marriage. No words were needed to tell them that we believed our child was God's most precious gift to us in our marriage. And, of course, we enjoyed showing her off, as any typical parents do!"

"Our small community held a turkey dinner one evening. My husband was working so I took our three year old and the baby. When we were being seated, the baby decided he was hungry. The room was packed and we were seated in the middle of a table of middle-aged and elderly people, most of whom I did not know. I knew he would either eat or cry, so I nursed him. Well, one woman filled my three-year-old's plate; another filled mine and even buttered my roll! The only comment was, 'It's so nice to see mothers nursing again.' We all had a wonderful meal and visit.

When our first child was 2½ years old, we flew to California to visit an aunt who never had children. Her home had white carpeting in one room, and beautiful breakable things throughout the house. During the visit we ate in restaurants unaccustomed to small children and visited homes of friends with grown children. Although I was somewhat apprehensive about how the visit would go, I knew I'd rather stay home than leave our child. Well, the trip was a success. Sara loved everything, was well behaved, and we received many compliments on her behavior. We let her know what to expect and how to act in each situation, and she really did well.

Our priest and members of our church commented on how well she acted in church. I believe this is partly because I've always taken her to church, and church is one place I expect her to be very, very quiet. If I left her at home or in a nursery until she was two or three or four, then brought her into church, it would be a difficult adjustment.

Looking back, I have never regretted taking my children anywhere. The only regrets and worry I felt were when I left my children and went out alone. I taught school the first year of parenting. Everyone told me over and over that I had the 'ideal' situation. I worked short hours, and went to Grandma's to nurse the baby at noon, and I got a break away from my baby. But for me, it was a terrible year. I never felt I was having a break. My heart was not in my work, but at home. Now I'm home full-time and I wouldn't trade my position with anyone. I take my children with me everywhere and I enjoy it. I have a friend who cannot shop with her two children because they won't behave. Instead of taking them along to show them how to act, she always leaves them at home. They'll never learn how to shop sitting at home, but only through experiencing it. As I look back over my experiences, I can't help but think of the advice I'd like to give other parents: Please take your children with you. They need to experience different situations, not a babysitter."

"I weaned the three older boys at seven months, three months, and eight months because my husband was always anxious for me to wean and get back to helping more with the ranch work. But baby #4 is with me constantly and she has experienced many things. We farmed together in a big Allis Chalmers tractor, we check heifers in the middle of the night during calving, and we rode a horse or two and moved some cows. She loves to cook and has her own little mixer so she can work along side me. In truth, I never left her for more than two hours until she was weaned at 26 months. My periods returned at 26 months postpartum. She had been nursing frequently until about a month previous.

When my girl was 18 months old, I was planning a visit to my 92-year-old grandmother. She called and said that she thought I'd better wean, because the baby was too old to be nursing and she needed to learn some independence. Likewise, she thought I needed to get on with my life, leave her behind so I could go places and do things on my own. I have to say that it upset me a lot, but I asked the Lord to show me His way. A few hours later when I took lunch to my husband in the hay, I told him what had been said and asked him if he thought I should wean her. With a tender look he said, 'No. You two are doing just fine!' If that is not a beautiful example of God changing a heart through prayer and perseverance, I don't know what is!"

"My husband is a pastor so we have many outside obligations to fulfill. We take our seven-month-old baby everywhere and when she is hungry or needs pacifying, I am there with her. Regarding breastfeeding, I was amazingly alone in my decision to do this. Even so-called 'progressive' mothers rely on formula and/or pacifiers. But I have found great support in women of my grandmother's age."

"Thank you for all the good articles on breastfeeding and natural child spacing. We have a healthy two year old who was raised on the advice of your magazine and book. She is still nursing, and it has been hard with a mother-in-law who thought she should have quit over a year ago. When our little girl was 14 months old, she was sick for four days with the flu. I kept nursing her afterwards, despite my mother-in-law's suggestions that it was the perfect time to wean her. After all the articles I'd read, I knew it wasn't. She is gradually weaning herself. And I will be sorry to see her quit because the nursing has been really relaxing for me. I think my mother-in-law has finally adjusted to my natural mothering."

"My third child had always been a difficult nurser. I nursed him anytime he wanted. At 16 months we rid him of his pacifier and nursing became a joy. From personal experience of nursing both culturally and ecologically, the difference is night and day for both baby and me. Ecological breastfeeding definitely made me feel closer to my baby."

"I enjoy receiving your magazine as I grow with my ten month old. As a newborn my daughter slept in a crib next to my bed. She had projectile vomiting for three months so I was afraid to let her sleep in the bed with us all night until later. After months of waking to her cries for nighttime nursing and bringing her to bed, I finally just started her out in our bed and what a difference. When she awakes at night and needs comforting, she can just roll over and nurse for as long as she likes while I snooze! Daddy loves having her in bed also as it has really made them closer.

I would encourage all new mothers to attend La Leche League meetings, at least once, before the birth of their child and read their manual, *The Womanly Art of Breastfeeding*. This book has been invaluable to me from before the birth of my daughter until now. I don't know how many times I referred to it when everyone kept telling me to use a pacifier, put my baby in bed and let her cry it out, and use other unnatural practices which are widely accepted by our society. I thank the Lord that I had my CCL teacher and dear friend to help me through those first unsettling months of motherhood. Support is the most important thing for a first-time mother."

"Our son is a gift from God. Some of the happiest times with him have been nursing him following the ecological breastfeeding guidelines. He was 18 pounds by his four-month checkup, though at birth he was only six pounds. My husband and I are very thin and everyone jokes that he's not ours. They are even more surprised when we say he just nurses. It's been so easy and enjoyable to nurse him at night in our bed. He's a very contented baby and has brought us a lot of happiness."

"It is such a good feeling to know that I can give my baby something that no one else can. It is also good to know that through nursing I can express my love for her even when I'm terribly upset at her. When I sit down and nurse her, I become calm again. I really believe that nursing helped me to become more patient with her and to be willing to take time out just to play or cuddle even if the dishes aren't done and the floor needs mopping. I was 'lucky' not to have the 'advantage' of popping a bottle into her mouth and to have an excuse to leave everything behind and enjoy the quiet time of nursing.

It is hard to believe how education about natural mothering has changed my outlook. Two years ago I would have never thought I would still be nursing at 15 months, nor would I have considered sharing our bed with the baby. Thanks to people like you and La Leche League, I'm growing more and more into the mother I should be."

"I have never given my baby a bottle and don't plan to. Since reading your book, I've taken her off rice cereal and baby food which made her constipated anyway. My husband and I plan to take her with us to Key West, Florida on a trip my husband earned through his job. I am so thankful that he supports me in the breastfeeding and understands why I can't leave her home during that trip, even with the most trusted caregivers."

"What saddens me is that in four years, I have met only one person who nursed as long as 15 months. My two sisters weaned their babies at three and six months. I have no support from family or friends. They do not understand why I would want to be 'tied down' and seem to think I'm somehow nursing 'so long' for myself, either to keep him dependent on me, or insinuating that I get some sort of thrill from it! I truly believe that I am doing what is best for my baby. My husband does respect and support me and says I'm the best mother in the world."

"Nursing lying down saved me. I was tired and tense, and I couldn't relax enough to nap. The solution: I nursed lying down after lunch. The baby fell asleep and the nursing hormones relaxed me enough to allow me to sleep. We're still nursing at 13 months postpartum and no menstruation yet."

167

"Natural mothering has brought me to a deeper understanding of God and how incredible He is. I now see that there is a divine plan for those trusting in Him. I love my children more and now look at them as a gift. I was brought up to get away from the children, and I did ignore mine a lot. It seemed wrong to do this; but being brought up this way in modern society, I was and am inclined toward this behavior. Thanks for teaching me so much."

"I want you to know what ecological breastfeeding and natural mothering has taught me. I've learned it helps squash the selfishness that our world tells us we deserve. The phrases 'my time' and 'my space' could not be in my vocabulary. As long as I stayed focused on God and His will for me and kept the world's view shut tightly out of my mind, I was at peace with myself and my daughter. But as soon as I let that world's door crack open even slightly, the peace began to erode.

I remember once thinking that I had to wean her. I went over in my mind all the things I had heard from other mothers — I have to go to my husband's office party and can't take the baby... I can't sleep because I am afraid of crushing her... I can't stand for someone always needing me...I need some time alone... I need my own space... I have to have some peace and quiet in the evening... I need to be able to go out with my friends... I don't like it when people think I am strange...

I suddenly realized that all those statements started with 'I'! What about the baby? If anyone asked my baby what she wanted and needed, she would probably say: I need my mom to hold me and cuddle me when I cry, and I don't even know why I cry sometimes but it feels better when she holds me... I need my mom's milk for sustenance, but sometimes even more for comfort... I feel so afraid when I am alone in that big cold bed in the dark room, and just the touch and smell of my mom's skin helps me rest... I like being with my mom and seeing all kinds of new things... I don't really understand why my mom leaves sometimes and those other people try to take care of me...

Of course, these are just my thoughts, but how often do we ponder these things in our hearts? We are so quick to accept the ways of the world and look at everything from a ME perspective! I am grateful that natural mothering has made me more aware of the needs of my children and conquered some of the selfish spirit that this world instills in me."

"Your book has helped me by validating my efforts and is priceless for the encouragement it offers, especially in dealing with unsolicited advice from people who tell us, "You're spoiling the baby!" I wonder how the human race has survived when a two-week-old baby is considered 'spoiled' if picked up when she cries. We would be a healthier race if all mothers responded to their babies' cries and if schedules, pacifiers, and cribs were never invented."

"In looking back, I would embrace the practice of natural mothering all over again for each baby. I fondly reflect on all the times I gazed down at my nursing child with awe and great love. I thank God for such a perfect arrangement for mother and baby to bond and nurture one another. At times I reflect on what it would have been like to have bottlefed my babies and left them with sitters frequently. I'm sure our life would have been different, but certainly not better. I praise God for showing me His mothering plan and natural family planning from the start of our marriage."

The Ecology of Natural Mothering

Our attention is often drawn toward the science of ecology and its importance in developing a better world for tomorrow. Man is learning that there is a balance in nature and that when he interferes with this balance, there can be some serious side effects. The environmentalists express their concerns about some issues that affect each one of us, such as: 1) quality of life for the child, 2) quality of life for the mother, 3) pollution, and 4) population. However, who among them have stressed breastfeeding as an ecological issue? In all four areas our environment could be improved by heeding that most basic form of ecology between mother and baby — breastfeeding. Ecological breastfeeding has many advantages, not only for mother and baby, but also for the wider environment in which we live.

Quality of life for the child

Dr. Otto Schaefer studied what happens when man, in this case the Eskimos, adopt the commerce-sponsored methods of infant feeding. He found that the bottlefed Eskimo children had a higher incidence of gastrointestinal diseases, respiratory diseases and middle-ear diseases, and anemia compared to the traditionally breastfed youngsters. Chronic ear infections, he said, were a very common health problem among bottlefed children. In addition, he states: "Changing infant nutrition practices and the extraordinary perversion of the female breast from a nutritional organ to a sex symbol, which is so typical in Western civilization, has affected the individual's health far beyond infancy, as the markedly higher incidence of allergic and auto-immune diseases in bottlefed than in breastfed children suggests."[1] In many areas of the world where bottlefeeding is a common practice, the health protection afforded the baby through breastfeeding has been eliminated.

Can babysitters and daycare affect the child emotionally? We now know that a child can suffer according to the degree of maternal deprivation he experiences during the first few years of life. He may receive the best of physical care with respect to his body, but if he lacks a mother or consistent mother-substitute he does not have the best start in life. An infant thrives on love, security, and intimacy from his mother. By being held, cuddled, and kept in frequent touch with his mother, the child has a richer start than the child who is left with many babysitters or is allowed to spend hours in an area without the close presence of his mother. Breastfeeding naturally helps to keep the mother close to her baby and ensures this type of care.

An American mother wrote me to explain how she became impressed with a form of natural mothering that she had not witnessed in her own country:

> As a college student I majored in intercultural studies and realized many of our child-rearing practices did not seem as successful for either mother or child as those in many non-Western countries, at least in their traditional cultures. I traveled in Africa one summer, and, even though a baby of my own was the farthest thing from my mind, I couldn't help but notice how happy and content all the babies and small children seemed, though I'm certain the general nutrition of their families was usually inadequate. The babies were almost always carried on their mother's backs and children and mothers were together. These facts stayed with me and influenced my attitudes toward our family.

In societies where mother and baby are separate, the rationalization that crying is good for a baby seems to be common. Amazingly and erroneously, some self-styled experts even dare to say that it is normal for a baby to cry one to three hours daily! Such crying did not occur in our home. But this philosophy of letting babies cry is a popular Western practice in caring for babies. For analyses of such erroneous trends today, you are welcome to view the parenting page of the CCL website.[2]

Dr. Lee Salk and Rita Kramer discussed this aspect of child raising in their book, *How To Raise A Human Being*.

> There's no harm in a child crying: the harm is done only if his cries aren't answered. Babies who are left to cry for long periods of time and are overwhelmed by frustration develop neurotic behavior, in extreme cases even become psychotic. If you ignore a baby's signal for help, you don't teach him independence. How can a helpless infant be independent? What you teach him is that no other human being will take care of his needs.[3]

Breastfeeding may reduce child abuse. For one thing, the mother is there to protect her baby or child from others. Just as important, I believe that breastfeeding can bring a change for the better within the mother. One mother told me that she had spanked each of her breastfed children only once or twice, yet she often spanked her bottlefed children when they were younger. She felt she had a greater sensitivity toward her breastfed children. Another mother said she felt she would be much rougher with her child if she didn't breastfeed. Other mothers breastfeed only because they do not want their children to grow up with the type of distant mothering that they received. They believe also that breastfeeding will help them in their mothering. God knows that parenting can be difficult. That's why He gives us prolactin, the motherly hormone that is released by nursing. This hormone helps breastfeeding moms to feel more motherly.

Mothers also notice changes in their children's behavior or their parenting behavior once they decide to try the natural mothering program or its associated philosophy of being in tune to their child's needs. One friend said when they sought counseling for their ten-year-old son, the first thing the counselor suggested before they tried to determine the cause of the problem was for the parents to have the child sit in their laps or to rock him. She found her son's behavior improved immediately with this kind of physical contact. The following true examples illustrate the need for children to have this special physical loving closeness with their mother.

> Our son is in the terrible-two stage at this time and we seem to be always yelling and spanking him. The past two days I have catered to his wants totally, and my husband remarked how affectionate and well behaved he seemed to be and asked jokingly if he were sick. He is not aware of my reading your book or a change in my attitude. Things go much smoother now, even though I am doing what others would consider spoiling him.

> I wanted to say that from my experience as a daughter and mother, natural mothering is the only way to raise children. My father (a doctor) never let my mother get close to me for fear of having a momma's baby, even telling her to give up nursing since I cried more often than every three hours. I feel that idea has hurt our relationship today. I am not able to be open to them and confide in them.
>
> As a mother at 19, I tried to follow the typical advice about formulas and schedules and potty training, and became a very frustrated mother to the point of shaking and spanking my child. After four more babies I gradually changed. I nursed the last one and really learned how to enjoy all of them. As for my parents, they were ready to pack their bags and go home once when I tried to rock and hold our eight year old while she was having a temper tantrum. Thanks for listening.

Breastfeeding provides a wonderful opportunity for physical contact between mother and baby. For those parents who fear they may hurt their children physically or abuse them verbally and become excessively angry with their children, breastfeeding is an excellent way to learn patience and strive to be that better parent.

For mothers or fathers who find they have repeatedly abused their children with regard to discipline, counseling may help. If you want to get a picture of what it is like to be abused physically or verbally by your parent, I highly recommend reading *The Man Who Listens to Horses* by Monty Roberts.[4] His father's pain-based techniques of horse training and child rearing led his son to look for a better way, so he learned how to create an atmosphere of trust in training horses and in raising children without violence. In his book he compares the environment in which a horse learns to the environment in which children learn. Monty and his wife took in many difficult foster children in the pre-teen and teen years. As Monty said: "Humans have said to horses *you do what I tell you or I'll hurt you.* Humans still say that to each other, still threaten and force and intimidate." I have never ridden a horse, but I found this book fascinating in content and in its relation to raising children. For parents who have tendencies similar to Mr. Roberts' dad, this best-seller book may be helpful.

In other cultures where breastfeeding is common, it is noted that the mother does not hit her child, and yet she disciplines. A *National Geographic* article described a society in which affection is the permeating force and violence is lacking; it noted that the women breastfed for several years and that mothers are firm when disciplining their children but do not spank them.[5]

In the oneness relationship found in breastfeeding, how can the mother strike or be violent with her child? It is as unlikely as a mother who would strike or mishandle herself. Lucky indeed is the child who is nursed for several years, for his mother will probably have a close relationship with him, and hopefully that closeness will remain even after the breastfeeding days are gone.

The importance of a mother's loving touch has been revealed especially in some difficult cases where it has apparently resulted in startling improvements in the child's behavior. In one case, a baby approached death as his blood sugar level dropped to zero soon after childbirth. With emergency care he survived, but it was believed that brain damage had occurred. The parents, however, were encouraged by their doctor who explained that with the best of care the brain, especially of a newborn, could be reprogrammed.

After a two-week stay in the hospital, the baby — who would just lie there and who lost almost all the responses normal to a small baby — was allowed to come home. Even though he sucked poorly from the bottle filled with breastmilk, the mother gradually taught him to nurse at the breast. But what is most impressive is the beautiful care this baby was fortunate enough to receive. The mother said:

> In addition to the breastfeeding, David always slept with me and was constantly carried, either in my arms or in a baby carrier on my chest. Every evening, after the children were in bed, I would take off all his clothes and play with him, caressing every part of his body, particularly his head. He also had a leisurely bath each morning, during which there was a great deal of physical contact. Gradually he began to respond and cry and react like a normal baby.[6]

Upon pediatric examination and neurological testing at five months of age, the child, who had been fed on mother's milk only, was found to be completely normal, and there was no evidence of permanent brain damage.

The specialists could not believe that this was the same child who had been so sick as a newborn.

Does nature have the answer to childcare? It may be worth a try. More writers are stressing the importance of the first few years of life, the importance of the mother-baby relationship, the importance of the mother responding to her baby's cries or fussiness and loving him dearly without fear of spoiling him. Going contrary to the culture, they stress that many babies or young children did not receive enough cuddling and holding. Some experts now believe that children who are having behavioral problems in school lacked touching or stimulation when necessary for normal development. Frances Cress Welsing, a Washington, D.C. psychiatrist, claims that many children receive "too little lap time"; she believes that little ones suffer when their mothers work or are too busy to take the time to hold them and thus their emotional needs are not met.[7]

More institutions are recognizing the importance of touching in caring for the sick and even the dying. Some institutions practice an individualized treatment of loving care, especially for special children. I was privileged to witness this type of care among the non-ambulatory, profoundly handicapped children at St. Joseph's Infant and Maternity Home in Cincinnati where one of our daughters was a volunteer. When the nun told the histories of these children and how they outlived their predicted life span for their particular illness, you knew where the answer lay. The volunteers were assigned to one child only and upon each visit spent two hours with his or her child. Most of the two hours was spent holding the young resident in one's lap or offering personal stimulation by loving and touching. During the summer months, the volunteers held his child in the outdoor pool, as these children loved water. Smiles were commonly observed on the faces of the staff and volunteers. Love permeated this "home." How much better this world would be if all children could receive this same type of wonderful care from their own parents, especially during their formative years.

Natural mothering is natural nurturing. It provides this same constant responsive care when a mother is always with her baby, nursing frequently and responding to his needs and accomplishments with lots of love. Breastfeeding is an excellent way for a little one to receive lots of lap time, cuddling, and touching in a positive, loving environment. The support and loving care of dad toward his wife and child is also invaluable to the child's emotional development.

Quality of life for the mother

A mother's own health also benefits from breastfeeding. The breastfeeding mother reduces her chance of developing breast cancer; the greater the number of children nursed and the longer the nursing period, the more protection is afforded. Breastfeeding is the natural method of releasing the placenta after birth. A nursing mother does not usually experience the "after-childbirth blues" unless she has to leave her baby to go back to work.

Nor will she experience a similar fate later under the natural weaning program since the hormonal changes occur very gradually.

Do women want reduced risk of ovarian cancer and reduced risk of premenopausal breast cancer? Then they should breastfeed. Do women want "improved bone remineralization postpartum with reduction in hip fractures in the postmenopausal period?" Then they should breastfeed. Do women want "less postpartum bleeding" and "a more rapid uterine involution?" Then they should breastfeed. Do women want to return to their prepregnant weight earlier? Then they should breastfeed. Do women want an increase in child spacing due to a delayed return of ovulation? Then they should breastfeed. All of these proven benefits are listed in the American Academy of Pediatrics' Policy Statement on Breastfeeding.[8]

In a few cases breastfeeding may even prevent surgery. One such lucky mother from Australia wrote:

> I suffered a third-degree prolapse of the uterus after the birth of our fourth child. The doctor suggested at only three weeks, then again at six weeks, after birth that I arrange immediately for surgery. I declined on the grounds that it would force weaning onto the baby as well as upset the general family balance. When he saw my reason was genuine, he agreed with my course of action and told me to grin and bear it as long as I could. Well, after four weeks the symptoms ceased to be hurtful and I gradually forgot its presence. At 10 months I had occasion to have another doctor do an examination of the cervix. Out of curiosity I asked for his comment on the prolapse; it turned out to be virtually disappeared. He heartily agreed with my suggestion that breastfeeding was the main help in restoring the sagging sinews and muscles to original condition.

It is a well known fact that nursing often after childbirth is nature's way of contracting the uterus back to its original size. The shots or pills given for this purpose are normally not necessary for the alert nursing mother.

It is also known that women have a higher iron requirement due to their monthly menstruation. Television ads frequently encourage women to take iron pills to maintain health and energy. Again, with good nutrition and natural mothering, the need for these pills would be greatly reduced. Through the prolonged absence of menstruation following childbirth, a woman regains her bodily store of iron which would otherwise be lost through her menstrual flow. As usual, if we look to nature we will find an answer, and certainly lactation amenorrhea has health benefits to the mother in her childbearing years.

Another physical aspect that is often forgotten in our busy world is the tranquilizing effect that nursing has on a woman. It provides brief rests during the day, and this form of relaxation can be a "plus factor" for the mother who tends to be tense and nervous. Breastfeeding is a good beginning for the mother as she feels satisfied in her new role and feels fulfilled in what she is doing.

Unfortunately many women are encouraged to seek fulfillment outside the home and to believe that fulfillment comes from doing it all — marriage, career, and children — simultaneously. Taking time out from the business or professional world to raise children is not a goal promoted by our society.

How did we arrive at this situation? Mothers wanted to be free to do more things and go more places. The bottle allowed them to leave their babies. The baby became less and less happy, and soon caregivers were resorting to more and more toys and equipment to entertain the baby while mother was being entertained or seeking fulfillment elsewhere. Others rationalized this mother-baby separation by the "crying-it-out" theory and the stated belief that it is normal for the baby to cry x-number of hours a day.

What has developed is a society in which parents go out of their homes, completely disregarding the fact that they are parents. Go to any women's or mothers' clubs or organizations (except groups that promote the natural, such as childbirth or breastfeeding) and you will rarely find a mother with her baby. Yet, if mothers read what is being written today, they should have their babies with them regardless of the method of feeding. I might add that the first couple we knew who took their baby with them to all social gatherings (in this case it was faculty gatherings) were bottlefeeding parents. Their baby was an especially good baby. Credit is due to their parenting. This was in 1970 and I was deeply impressed with this couple's commitment to parenting.

Bottlefeeding deprives a woman of the satisfactions and pleasures she should gain from breastfeeding. Bottlefeeding increases the chances of health problems for her baby. Her baby will probably be less intelligent than if he had received the brain-developing benefits of breastmilk. Bottlefeeding takes away the natural infertility designed for the mother by nature, and it allows the mother to set goals to leave her baby. On the other hand, breastfeeding makes separation painful, and a mother does all she can to avoid leaving her baby. This natural care also teaches the woman to give of herself totally to her baby, and this is one reason why the mother does not want to delegate the baby care to another person. I found that the more natural I became in my mothering, the more I kept my baby with me. We became as one.

Breastfeeding can affect parenting styles in later years. Let's take the problem of helping a child get to sleep. In a bottlefeeding society it is common to hear of parents using strict schedules or procedures for bedtime or naptime, strict words, bribes such as candy, and even medication. A neighborhood child once came to my door asking for aspirin, which he said his mother used to get them to go to sleep! Of course, I did not provide the aspirin. Some parents use the TV screen or music to put the children to sleep. Some parents put forth lots of effort and time to get their children to sleep at such-and-such a time.

With natural mothering children tend to sleep when they are sleepy. The giving of self usually continues by lying down with the child, rubbing his back, rocking him, singing some soft songs, and so on. The approach tends to be a continuation of the mother or the father giving of herself or himself.

Needless to say, much of the happiness in life and in parenting also comes from the giving. Too many women today tend to be too concerned about their careers or outside accomplishments or hobbies at the expense of their husbands, families, the unborn, and the young baby or children at home. Personal fulfillment is the ultimate goal. With breastfeeding, however, I feel that a woman learns that true fulfillment comes in the giving and not the taking. Being human, we all have to work at developing certain virtues, even when breastfeeding. No one is naturally good or loving. Most of us have a tendency to think mostly of ourselves. It is a continual job to put ourselves at the service of others and to develop better traits. Breastfeeding helps a mother to mature and to develop as a more-giving person in a very gradual and easy manner. Breastfeeding cannot guarantee that our children will turn out well, but it can become a learning process whereby a new mother begins to think of others, especially her children, and to develop certain caring virtues that can aid her during her later mothering years.

Pollution

Environmentalists should take an interest in advocating breastfeeding since it does not contribute to the pollution of our air or water, nor does it detract from the environment. Bottlefeeding involves the throwing away of certain items such as bottles, bottle liners, nipples, pacifiers, baby jars, cereal containers, sterilizers, formula cans, bottle brushes, and so forth. In addition, bottlefeeding entails the use of fuel and water in the preparing, heating, or sterilizing of the milk or food and the cleaning of the equipment to be used.

In our affluent society, we commonly observe the discarding of good clothes. Clothes that could be mended with a good patch or new zipper are simply thrown in the trash. With bottlefeeding a considerable number of good baby clothes and bibs are likely to be discarded if the baby or older child is given juice or fruit. Juices stain baby clothes so that they are soon unpresentable and are not worn again. With an exclusively breastfed baby, no clothes are stained. You can dress your baby up for a special occasion without worrying about food stains ruining the outfit. One mother claimed breastfeeding is ecologically best for her clothes too. She noted that her bottlefed babies ruined her good clothing when they spit up milk — it left a bad smell, but her breastfed babies' milk wiped off easily without leaving a bad smell. She enjoyed not having to wash or dry clean her clothes as frequently as in the past.

With natural breastfeeding there would also be some decrease in the usage of sanitary pads since mothers would be averaging over a year without menstruating after childbirth. Likewise, there would be a decrease in sales of bottle-related items, which would lower their production and thus decrease the amount of pollution connected with such production. There is no doubt that natural breastfeeding could have a favorable impact toward a better tomorrow from an environmental standpoint.

Other couples carry their interest in ecological breastfeeding to the wider area of natural family planning. One nursing mother who identified herself as not being affiliated with any religious group wrote:

> The reason that I am greatly enthused about natural family planning and will use it to the exclusion of any artificial method of contraception is not because of religious or moral reasons but because of health reasons. Artificial contraception is yet another way of pollution. It pollutes the body just as our city water and air, the many additives in our foods and bottlefeeding do. You are aware of the fact that with the ecology movement more and more people are becoming interested in antipolluting ways of living in every form possible. Birth control will be no exception. Let's hope that eventually natural family planning will be used by all those interested in keeping themselves, and the future generations, as pure as possible.

Population

More attention should be given to the role that ecological breastfeeding can play in the birthrate of an individual couple. The decline in breastfeeding is an important factor in increased birthrates, while the presence of breastfeeding is a key factor in the low birthrates of some primitive peoples.

A neighbor, upon watching a TV special on the Tasadays in the Philippines, was anxious to come over and tell me how long they breastfed their children and how the research people were amazed at their low birthrate. She, of course, immediately suspected that breastfeeding played a big factor in the low birthrate because the children are nursed into their early childhood. These were the same people referred to earlier in this chapter as having an absence of violence in their lives.

Dr. Otto Schaefer, a Canadian doctor, found the same relationship between shortened lactation and the population increase in some countries. He found this to be true among the Eskimos where prolonged lactation of about three years traditionally kept their family size small. He also found that the availability of bottles and formula at the trading posts changed their fertility patterns immensely.

> As something of a diversion while I was in Baffin Island in the mid-1950s, I made calculations that indicated that the intervals between siblings shrank in direct relation to the mileage of the family from the trading posts. The shorter the distance, the more frequently they had children. The effect of rapid development of communications and the consequent movements of former camp Eskimos into large settlements is reflected in the more-than-50% jump in the Eskimo birthrate in the Northwest Territories alone, and the increase from less than 40 births per 1,000 in the mid-1950s to 64 per 1,000 ten years later. In fact, it is seldom realized that in the last 20 years the Eskimos' population explosion has been as great as or greater than that which has occurred in any developing nation in the world. This is due less to the reduction in infant mortality than to the jump in birthrate. And it is far more intense for the urbanized Eskimo than for those who still live in the scattered hunting camps. There is a clear relationship between the increasing use of bottlefeeding and the shortening of lactation. This important point is usually overlooked in searches for explanations of the population explosion seen in developing countries.[9]

Dr. J. A. Hildes and the same Dr. Schaefer conducted some fascinating studies on the Igloolik Eskimos. The one outstanding observation dealt with the difference in the fertility rates among the older women as opposed to the younger women due to the changes in mothering practices. Women aged 30 to 50 years who had traditionally breastfed for two to three years conceived 20 to 30 months after childbirth. Remember, that is when they conceived, not when they gave birth. The younger mothers under 30 years of age who bottlefed conceived 2 to 4 months after childbirth. These doctors noted that other researchers attributed the population explosion in other countries to a reduced mortality rate. However, the Iglooliks have had a population increase in spite of their high infant death rate. The doctors found that it is the rapid urbanization of these Eskimos during the twenty post-World War II years that is responsible for the increase in births, urbanization that brought rapid communication, and the rapid introduction of the baby bottle to these people. Thus they lost the natural population control that prolonged breastfeeding had previously given them.[10]

Dr. R. V. Short from Scotland has presented papers on the lactation phase of reproduction and has claimed that "throughout the world as a whole, more births are prevented by lactation than all other forms of contraception put together."[11] Dr. Peter Howie from the United Kingdom claimed that for many areas "breastfeeding offered more protection than all methods of contraception combined." In his talk at the Fourth National and International Symposium on Natural Family Planning, Dr. Howie added one fascinating research statistic. Even when breastfeeding offered only 4 to 8 months of infertility, it has been demonstrated that breastfeeding still provided 31½ million couple-years of infertility. This means that 31½ million couples did not conceive in a single year due to breastfeeding. This is greater protection than all the unnatural forms of birth control (condoms, IUDs, pills, etc.) put together which was estimated at 24 million couple-years of fertility "protection." Howie is convinced that the population increased drastically during the last 500 years because of wet nursing, artificial baby milk and baby food.[12]

Natural mothering isn't going to cure all the world's problems, even in our personal families. But in this chapter I have tried to show its far reaching effects in our families and in the world at large. At the family level, it contributes to the physical and emotional health of both mother and baby. Also breastfeeding families tend to do things together, and stronger families make stronger societies. At the larger community level, it results in less pollution in a number of ways. At the level of both the individual family and the world, it provides a natural form of birth regulation. With all this going for natural mothering via the breast, it would seem more than appropriate that breastfeeding, and especially ecological breastfeeding, should be encouraged at all levels.

[1] Otto Schaefer, "When the Eskimo Comes to Town," *Nutrition Today*, November/December 1971.

[2] CCL website: www.ccli.org.

[3] L. Salk and R. Kramer, *How to Raise a Human Being*, New York: Random House, 1969.

[4] Monty Roberts, *The Man Who Listens to Horses*, New York: Random House, 1997.

[5] Kenneth MacLeish and John Launois, "The Stone Age Men of the Philippines," *National Geographic*, August 1972.

[6] Donald Parker, "David's Story," *La Leche League News*, March-April 1971.

[7] William Raspberry, "Preventing Some Social Ills," *The Cincinnati Enquirer*, July 1, 1985.

[8] American Academy of Pediatrics, "Policy Statement: Breastfeeding and the Use of Human Milk," *Pediatrics*, December 1977, 1035-39.

[9] Schaefer, op. cit.

[10] J. Hildes and O. Schadfer, "Health of Igloolik Eskimos and Changes with Urbanization," Paper presented at the Circumpolar Health Symposium, Oulu, Finland, June 1971.

[11] R. Short, "The Evolution of Human Reproduction," *Proc. R. Soc. Lond.*, 195(1976), 3-24.

[12] P. Howie, "Synopsis of Research on Breastfeeding and Fertility," *Breastfeeding and Natural Family Planning*, Bethesda, Maryland: KM Associates, 1986, 7-22.

20

Disappointments with Natural Mothering

Mothers who complain about ecological breastfeeding generally fall into two categories: 1) those who believe they followed the program but had an early return of menstruation, and 2) those who want another baby but are still infertile due to the breastfeeding. In the former situation, the mother feels the natural mothering program did not "work" for her, while in the latter situation the program "works" too well and a desired pregnancy seems impossible at the present time.

"It doesn't work"

Our first concern will be those mothers who have an unexpected early return of their periods. The first thing to remember is that the primary purpose of ecological breastfeeding is to provide optimum care and nutrition for your baby. Extended infertility is a normal *side* effect. Second, every study shows a *range* in the return of fertility after childbirth. If the average return of fertility is 15 months, 50% of returns will be less than 15 months and 50% will be more than 15 months. Third, if you have a very early return of fertility, that may be nature's plan for you. Fourth, regardless of when your fertility returns, you can detect its return and switch into systematic natural family planning using the several fertility awareness signs.

Hospital restrictions

Some breastfeeding experts have wondered if hospital restrictions on breastfeeding may interfere with breastfeeding infertility. These restrictions come at a very critical time in the establishment of breastfeeding amenorrhea. Mothers should insist on unrestricted nursing from childbirth on or choose a hospital or birthing center that promotes mother-baby togetherness and unlimited nursing.

Fatigue

Another factor that may interfere with breastfeeding is fatigue. I am convinced that this is a time when a mother should slow down and be more involved with her baby, husband and family and not be overly involved with the world and outside activities. It's a time to just enjoy your baby. I'm not saying you should stop all involvement; however, outside activities should be minimal, and housework or activities should not cause excessive strain. Fatigue can hinder the milk supply and the letdown reflex. As one mother said, "I think my periods returned early from too much work during the canning season, and I didn't get enough rest." When fatigue sets in, pre-menstrual feelings may develop. Your body is sending you signals to slow down and get more rest. Why not get in a daily nap and adequate sleep at night before these feelings develop? If you have pre-menstrual feelings, nurse your baby during the daily nap and during the night. The added rest for you and the added nursing that occurs while you sleep may eliminate those pre-menstrual sensations.

Unfortunately, most mothers attempting ecological breastfeeding have not read this book. They have been going only by the information provided by the Couple to Couple League at its NFP classes, or through the CCL manual, or by hearsay. While the fourth edition of *The Art of Natural Family Planning* is more complete than previous editions, it has to be succinct. For example, it has two pages on nighttime and naptime nursing. This breast-feeding book has more than a chapter. Therefore, it seems that if a couple is truly interested in the spacing aspect of breastfeeding, they would want to read the only book on this subject. In a society where long-term lactation is the accepted practice for baby care, this latter recommendation would not be necessary. However in a bottlefeeding culture, reading this book is almost a necessity if a couple wants to provide the best care for their baby and desires extended natural postpartum infertility.

A very small percentage of women may still experience an early return of menstruation regardless of following the advice in this book. In general, if your baby is sleeping through the night, if you have reduced your nursings, or if you are leaving the baby for a length of time, then begin systematic natural family planning fertility awareness in anticipation of a probable early return of fertility.

A Checklist

"I had an early return of menstruation. Did I do the following?" The first list includes the obvious.

_____ Exclusive breastfeeding the first 6 months of life
_____ No pacifiers
_____ No bottles
_____ No solids during the first 6 months
_____ Nursed and slept with the baby during a daily nap
_____ Nursed and slept with the baby during the night
_____ Used frequent and unrestricted nursings
_____ Kept baby physically close to me

The following are situations that may be less applicable as possible causes of an early return of menstruation, but I list them for possible consideration.

_____ Baby had an illness and decreased his nursing.

_____ My reluctance to nurse often

_____ My reluctance to nurse modestly in front of others (i.e. visiting relatives)

_____ My reluctance to include the baby into our activities

_____ Absence of the family bed

_____ Absence of a daily nap

_____ Baby is not an eager or frequent nurser.

_____ I was fatigued for some reason.

Parents or professionals who are interested in promoting ecological breastfeeding may find this checklist helpful.

The summary checklist

The "Summary of Ecological Breastfeeding and Natural Child Spacing Program" is included in the first chapter of this book and is available at the CCL website and on a one-sided sheet from CCL headquarters. This "Summary" can be used to teach the Seven Standards of ecological breastfeeding. It also has a checklist to use for teaching and for analysis when a mother experiences an early return of menstruation.

"It works too well"

While many couples enjoy a long period of breastfeeding amenorrhea and infertility, it may become a source of frustration when the couple desires another baby. The nursing mother may try to eliminate a feeding or reduce the nursing by doing other activities with her child. Occasionally this helps, but often in the natural mothering process the child is not ready to skip a feeding, and tears roll down his face. It becomes quite evident through his behavior that he still has a real need to nurse, and to try to skip that nursing when he is tired before naptime or bedtime is almost impossible. With child-led weaning these feedings are gradually dropped when there is no longer a need, but many couples still experience frustration, or disappointment comes while waiting and waiting for the return of fertility. Some of these mothers are women who started having children later in life, and they see their reproductive years nearing an end.

A few couples will not be able to achieve pregnancy until after their child is completely weaned — even though they are having regular menstrual cycles and their chart shows the fertile signs and a strong postovulation thermal shift. Furthermore, the same woman who may be unable to become pregnant while nursing one baby can conceive easily while nursing another. One friend was nursing an almost-two-year-old and desired another baby. Her chart showed all the signs of fertility and she could not achieve pregnancy. Dr. Konald Prem, who helped us start the Couple to

Couple League, assured her she would get pregnant the first cycle after weaning. Eventually the child weaned and she did become pregnant the following cycle after weaning! I later met her at a conference, and she was nursing her third baby who was conceived while nursing her second child. Thus in her case, history did not repeat itself.

Most couples can look to a return of menstruation as a sign of future fertility if another baby is desired. But what happens if there is no return of menstruation? What are the feelings a couple is experiencing when they yearn for another baby but the mother is still in amenorrhea? A mother wrote about this particular problem in the CCL magazine, *CCL Family Foundations*:

> Our son will be three years old soon. Basically he nurses at nap, bed-times, the odd time through the night, and on a bad day for comfort. I have read the CCL manual and have been practicing natural family planning as much as I can. My menstruation has not yet resumed, so I began taking my temperature and observing any mucus and cervical signs, looking hopefully for ovulation in spite of having no period. However, my temperatures remain low. The cervix remains low, firm, and closed; and to date there is no sign of fertile mucus.
>
> All of this is unfortunately discouraging, as my husband and I wish to conceive again. I do hope for a return to fertility soon. I feel that any amount of sucking stimulation from my son is all that is necessary to suppress my ovulation. I'm sure I am on the long end of the scale for lactation amenorrhea. I do not wish to force weaning as I believe in allowing him to take the lead in his own development, but this does put me at odds — wanting to continue to meet my toddler's needs.
>
> Child spacing of three years is what I had hoped for, but it may extend to four years. I had enjoyed natural mothering immensely until recently and this, of course, is due to wanting another child.

The magazine received some excellent responses to this couple's dilemma. I'd like to share them with you. They provide different insights to this particular problem which may be helpful to others in a similar situation.

> I would like to share the experience of someone I know. The woman married and conceived in her early twenties. She weaned the baby at about one year due to cultural reasons. She could not conceive again until after six years when she conceived with the help of a fertility drug. She liked the idea of baby-led weaning, but when her 16-month-old was still nursing, she made the decision to wean so she could go back onto fertility drugs to achieve another pregnancy. She weaned her toddler (not too happily) and before she could begin the drugs, she discovered she was pregnant. With this baby she was relaxed and didn't worry about hurrying the weaning. But she discovered she was pregnant when the baby was a year old and this pregnancy turned out to be twins. Four children under the age of four are a handful. The situation made for a strained marital situation and strained economic situation. How different her situation may have been if she had listened to her second baby's need to nurse a

little longer. We never know what the future holds or what God has in store for us.

The three-year-old's mother has no guarantee that she will ever conceive again or that her second baby will not miscarry. If it turned out that this was your only child, would you regret having weaned him prematurely? Babies spaced four or even five years apart may not be what you planned, but consider that you are meeting the needs of your three-year-old who, after all, is only on loan from the Lord. If Jesus Himself had carried the baby to your front door and asked you to "take the best possible care of him," what would you do?

From a practical point of view, rejoice! You'll have the first child through college before the second child is there (not all bad). Take the best care you can of the child you have and trust in God for the children you hope for.

I always turn to your article first for support in my mothering style. My heart really went out to the mother who is nursing and wants to become pregnant. How discouraging to keep looking for fertility and discovering none. The difficult time can be depressing and makes it hard to enjoy the present time.

Take this special time in your son's life to enjoy him. Do other mothering activities such as trips to the park, reading, painting, etc., and you might notice your son's interest in nursing going down. If charting, please don't spend all your energy looking at the chart for long periods of time and fretting over it like I did.

Our four children were planned, but they never came in the exact month or even the year that they were longed for. I had to accept the fact that God is the Creator and it was difficult to accept, but the acceptance has caused my faith to grow in the long run.

I read an article in our local La Leche League newsletter about a mother with a nursing three year old. She was unable to conceive until her doctor advised her to gain 10 pounds which she did. She became pregnant within about three months after the weight gain without altering her nursing pattern. I have a close friend who is very thin (5'6" and about 108-110 lb.). She breastfed two children and menstruation did not return until after each was weaned. It is well known that anorexic women do not menstruate. Perhaps some women are borderline and a few nursings a day are enough to suppress their cycles.

In regard to the woman who was writing regarding her lactation amenorrhea, I think this can raise a question: Can a couple be selfish in wanting more children? I'm not saying this couple is, but I do think we need to trust God's design and timing more. If her fertility has not returned but her youngest still needs to nurse, this couple may want to seriously consider that the timing may not be right for another pregnancy yet. We planned our first child very deliberately but allowed God free reign with our second child. After 26 months of amenorrhea, I had four periods and conceived while charting laxly. If our baby had been born two weeks earlier or later, it would have been under extremely difficult circumstances.

As it was, God's timing was exquisite. It may be that more couples need to listen to the Lord more in guiding their family size and timing. It's food for thought and prayer anyway.

I experienced amenorrhea for two years and nine months while nursing my twin sons. I had anxiously awaited my period from about the time they turned two. I also thought a spacing of about three years would be nice. I did not encourage them to slow down the nursing. When my period returned, they were nursing before bedtime and naptime. I did have a few months warning that fertility was returning by signs of mucus. I felt elated when I discovered that I was pregnant after only one cycle. I figured my plan of three years apart would only be altered by six months. But then in my twelfth week of pregnancy I miscarried the baby. We were devastated. I felt like my whole life was just one big wait.

The next four months were miserable. My periods returned but they were erratic and ovulation was hard to pinpoint. Often my cycle was extra long and I would think I was pregnant again only to start a period on day 38 or 40. Finally I did become pregnant and delivered a healthy son when my older boys turned four. The child is now 20 months.

Now that it's over, the time it took to have another child seemed short. However, at the time I became consumed with the thoughts of pregnancy. I felt as if my body had played a cruel trick on me. Here I was doing what I thought was best for my sons by breastfeeding them, and, in a way, was being punished for it.

My conclusion has been to reconcile myself to God's will for us as a family. He has a divine plan for us and by allowing nature to do her thing I am not interfering with that plan. God's ways are not our ways. He knows what is best for us and understands our destiny. We can never fully appreciate this with our limited knowledge and must therefore trust in Him when things are not going as we would like. This can be hard to accept as I well know, but I also know how fallible my decisions can be. To think about it honestly, I'm relieved to let this important decision about spacing and consequently the number of children up to God. He knows what He is doing. The challenge is for us to accept and adjust to it in a positive way.

Sometimes it is nice to receive a follow-up letter to hear how events turned out after a mother has written. The mother who was nursing the three-year-old and desired another child wrote back, and this is what she had to say:

Thanks for your letter of support and encouragement earlier this year. Nature has taken its course. This past weekend when my son turned three years old, I had my first postpartum period. We are now back to recording temperature and fertility signs after giving it up for several months. I reread *Breastfeeding and Natural Child Spacing,* and a first postpartum period at 39 months was mentioned. I thought I would give myself at least that long, and it has happened.

I had been prepared for 18 to 24 months of amenorrhea, but three years seemed impossible. However, I feel it has proven best for our family. My son has always been a high need child and I'm sure he has needed all of this time alone. He is quite independent now and I feel he could accept my attention to a sibling. He would be about four years old when and if a new baby were to bless our family.

Our son still nurses at naptime and early evening before bedtime. I am sure the lack of night nursing is what finally allowed my hormonal system to return to normal cycles. I thought he was ready to wean, but he seemed to need his naptime nursing more than anything. Even when playing outside he'll stop play and tell me, "I need nappy. I need milky. Please, mommy." So we continue to enjoy this special time together. He is such a big boy in so many ways, but at this time he is still my baby who needs his mommy.

To think of nursing a toddler/child of this age would have been repulsive to me even when my first son was born; but having grown and evolved in this relationship together makes it so beautiful. Contact with La Leche League and the Couple to Couple League has given us needed support and encouragement.

These disappointments over an early return of menstruation or over an extended amenorrhea are mentioned to help others who find themselves in a similar situation. Those who have an unexpected early return may start charting for the return of fertility. For those couples who anxiously await another pregnancy, they can realize that God's plan for them does not include another baby at this time. In both situations, the woman is happier once she accepts her own natural pattern. Hopefully, the disappointment will only be temporary and the nursing mother will go on from there, accepting the unexpected gracefully and finding support from others and perhaps also from this chapter.

21

Personal Research

To test the theory that ecological breastfeeding spaces babies for American women just as it does for women in primitive and developing parts of the world, my husband and I conducted two studies, one in 1971 and another in 1986. In both studies the readers of the early editions of this book returned a survey about their recent breastfeeding experiences. In both studies we used the first postpartum menstruation or any form of spotting as an indication of the end of amenorrhea and the return of fertility. We realize that this is not the best determination of fertility; the temperature graph is far superior. Nevertheless, it provides a fairly accurate indicator and is universally applicable.

What we found in both studies confirmed our basic conviction that ecological breastfeeding provides significantly more postpartum infertility than cultural breastfeeding. The results showed that on the average babies will be spaced about two years apart with ecological breastfeeding, assuming random intercourse and no form of birth control and no use of systematic periodic abstinence.

The 1971 study

In this study we collected 112 nursing experiences from 72 mothers. Most of the experiences occurred before the mothers read this book.[1]

First, we found the average length of amenorrhea of the entire study group: 10.2 months. This included both cultural and ecological nursing experiences. Then we selected **six criteria for ecological breastfeeding**. These criteria are directly related to practices that increase or decrease the amount of suckling at the breast. You will notice that the criteria differ very little from the Seven Standards used today. In the past those criteria were:

1. No pacifiers used
2. No bottles used
3. No liquids or solids for five months
4. No feeding schedules other than baby's
5. Presence of night feedings
6. Presence of lying-down nursing for naps and night feedings.

Duration of amenorrhea

Our analysis showed that 29 of the entire 112 nursing experiences fulfilled all these requirements. In these 29, the mothers nursed 22.8 months on the average; this was 40% longer than the 16.3 months of nursing for the entire sample.

Of great significance, the ecological breastfeeding group **averaged 14.6 months of breastfeeding amenorrhea**, and this was 43% longer than the average of 10.2 months of amenorrhea experienced in the entire group.

Actually, the contrast between those doing ecological breastfeeding and those doing some form of cultural breastfeeding was greater than illustrated by these numbers because the figures for the "sample as a whole" included the ecological breastfeeding group. This inclusion raised the average for the sample as a whole, so in our 1986 study we directly compared the ecological breastfeeding experiences with those of the cultural breastfeeding experiences.

Early return of menstruation

There were only two cases of menstruation returning prior to seven months postpartum in our sample of 29 cases of natural mothering. One woman who engaged in the natural mothering program experienced the return of menstruation at six weeks postpartum. However, she kept basal temperature charts, which indicated infertile cycles up through the eleventh month postpartum. The second mother, whose menstruation returned at four months postpartum, also used basal temperature charts which indicated a return of ovulation six or seven months postpartum.

Conception prior to menstruation

In the entire group of 112 returned questionnaires, there were 14 instances of pregnancy occurring prior to the return of menstruation. The number who indicated that they were relying on amenorrhea for conception regulation was 89. Thirteen of these 14 provided enough detailed information for analysis of their baby care and feeding program. Of these 14 who became pregnant prior to menstruation, only two were among the 29 who followed the natural mothering program with its six criteria. One mother conceived at 27 months postpartum, but she had deliberately reduced her nursing in order to conceive; the other mother became pregnant at 15 months postpartum. The other 11 mothers were from the larger sample whose nursing habits were more typical of a bottlefeeding culture. An analysis in Table I indicates significant factors in their nursing, mothering, or feeding patterns.

There were no conceptions by any mother in the natural mothering group prior to the twelfth month, and the earliest conception without a "warning" menstruation was at 15 months as stated above.

Table I:
Relationship of nursing patterns to conception
during amenorrhea in eleven cultural nursing experiences

Month of conception	Comment
2nd	Began liquids on day 1, used pacifier
5th	Began liquids at 1 month, solids at 4 months, night feedings for only 3 months
6th	Began solids/liquids at 6 months, no night feeding
7th	Began solids at 3 months, liquids at 6 months, night feedings for only 3 months, nursed on a schedule, no lying-down nursing
8th	Solids at 2 months, liquids at 7 months, pacifier used
8th	Weaned at 8 months, conceived before period returned
9th	Exclusive nursing for 1 month, solids at 4 months (other data insufficient)
11th	Solids at 5 months (no other data)
11th	Solids at 4 months, liquids at 6 months, night feedings for 6 months, used pacifier
12th	Solids at 5 months
14th	Solids at 5 months, used bottle and pacifier, night feedings for 10 months

The 1986 study

During the next 15 years we accumulated over 1,500 breastfeeding surveys. Early in 1986 CCL Teaching Couple Oscar and Susan Staudt wrote a data analysis computer program, and a student nurse entered 286 surveys for analysis. The surveys used were not pre-selected, but the surveys from especially long amenorrheas had been filed separately and were not used. Using the same six criteria we used in 1971, we found 98 nursing experiences that qualified as ecological breastfeeding.[2]

Total months of breastfeeding

One of the biggest differences between the two surveys was the average duration of breastfeeding for the entire sample. In the 1986 study, the 286 nursing experiences averaged 20.4 months, 25% longer than the 16.3 average duration in the 1971 survey. We speculated that this increase may be due to two facts: 1) an increased social acceptance of more extended nursing; 2) reading the earlier edition of this book and the "natural mothering" columns in the newsletter of the Couple to Couple League may have motivated mothers to nurse longer.

Duration of amenorrhea

The average duration of amenorrhea for the 286 nursing experiences was 11.7 months compared with 10.2 in 1971. The sample of 98 ecological breastfeeding experiences averaged 14.5 months of amenorrhea. We think this was the most important finding of this study because it confirmed the primary finding of the 1971 study where we had found an average of 14.6 months of breastfeeding amenorrhea with ecological breastfeeding. We now have two studies 15 years apart yielding almost identical results on this key point, so we can say with greater confidence than before that women in a bottlefeeding culture who follow the pattern of ecological breastfeeding will average 14.5 months of amenorrhea.

Comparison between ecological and cultural breastfeeding

A comparison was made between the ecological breastfeeding group and the cultural breastfeeding experiences, and the results are illustrated in Table II. The total adds up to 284 experiences because two computer records failed to be tallied.

Table II:
Comparison of Duration of Amenorrhea

Ecological Breastfeeding
N = 98

Average Months of Nursing	25.7
Average Months of Amenorrhea	14.5

Cultural Breastfeeding
N= 186

Average Months of Nursing	17.5
Average Months of Amenorrhea	10.3

The ecological breastfeeding mothers averaged approximately 40% greater duration of amenorrhea than the cultural breastfeeding mothers.

We then tried to discover if there was any single one of the six criteria we used for ecological breastfeeding that by itself showed an even greater duration of amenorrhea, but we found none. Since we were unable to find any single factor which could be effective for 12 months or more, we were confirmed in our conviction that it is a combination of all the elements of natural mothering which results in the side effect of a year or more of natural infertility, on the average. Our research therefore confirms that it is the entire package of ecological breastfeeding that spaces babies. This form of baby care is the Creator's original form of natural family planning.

Variation and possible causes

Significant variation in the return of menstruation continued to be recorded among mothers doing ecological breastfeeding. Of these cases, 93% were in amenorrhea at six months, 56% were still in amenorrhea at one year, and 34% were still in amenorrhea at 18 months.

We do not know what causes this sort of variation. If two mothers are following the same breastfeeding pattern but one has a return of menstruation at six months and the other at 16 months, we don't know why — **if** both mothers are following the entire program. The checklist provided in Chapter 20 and the Summary provided in Chapter 1 may help those parents or professionals interested in the promotion and practice of ecological breastfeeding and child spacing.

Undoubtedly some of the variation in the length of amenorrhea can be attributed to the differences in the suckling needs and nursing patterns of different babies. In addition there are probably differences in the way bodies of different women respond to the same amount of suckling stimulus.

All past and current research dealing with breastfeeding infertility supports the basic thesis of this book: that ecological breastfeeding with its frequent and unrestricted suckling of the baby at the breast is nature's way of spacing babies.

[1] J. and S. Kippley, "The Relation Between Breastfeeding and Amenorrhea: Report of a Survey," *JOGN Nursing*, November/December 1972, 15-21.
[2] J. and S. Kippley, "The Spacing of Babies with Ecological Breastfeeding," *International Review*, Spring/Summer 1989, 107-116.

Natural Family Planning

Responses to the earlier editions of *Breastfeeding and Natural Child Spacing* included many requests for further information about systematic natural family planning (**NFP**). Many couples see a logical package that includes both forms of natural family planning — ecological breastfeeding and systematic NFP. With the former, you are doing what's best for the baby and strengthening the bond between mother and child; with the latter, you are doing what's best for the marriage and strengthening the bond between husband and wife.

Technological man has succeeded in his efforts to separate sex and procreation almost completely. Technology can give freedom from the risk of pregnancy, freedom to have unlimited sexual intercourse, freedom from carrying a child for nine months, and, of course, freedom from the old-fashioned mammalian activity called breastfeeding. My husband and I see natural family planning as the only real answer to the technological invasion of human sexuality, love and procreation.

Just as there has been much ignorance about breastfeeding both in general and with special reference to natural child spacing, so is there much ignorance about systematic natural family planning. Some say it is not reliable. That is a half-truth. Couples who are ill-informed or who choose to ignore the signs of fertility will have unforeseen pregnancies, but for couples who are well-informed and who live by what they know, systematic NFP is reliable and highly effective — at the 99% level. Even the less educated can learn this natural method with dedicated teachers. Mother Teresa informed my husband during a phone conversation that her nuns teach systematic NFP, either the mucus-only method or the temperature-only method, to people who have little or no formal education, people in the slums of Calcutta.

In the very beginning (1971), the Couple to Couple League taught couples systematic natural family planning and ecological breastfeeding. Soon the correspondence and personal witness of couples indicated that many couples not only learned about the natural methods of birth regulation but also were discovering that natural family planning strengthened their marriages. This was especially true for those couples who had used contraception. Some couples have told us that NFP "saved" their marriage. From the limited data available to us, it appears that couples using natural family planning have a divorce ratio of not over 5% (1 divorce for every 20 marriages) and maybe as low as 2% (1 divorce for every 50 marriages) compared to contracepting couples who have a divorce ratio in the area of 50% (1 divorce for every 2 marriages).

Of particular importance for the nursing mother in determining the return of fertility is the observation of cervical mucus and/or the cervix itself. As we noted in an earlier chapter, the available evidence indicates that about 94% of nursing mothers with babies six months or older will experience menstruation before achieving pregnancy. To find out if she is in that small group for whom fertility comes before her first menstruation, the nursing mother can examine herself and chart her signs of fertility or infertility. This is all well explained in *The Art of Natural Family Planning*, the users' manual of the Couple to Couple League.

Suffice it to say that the well-informed mother can detect the onset of fertility before her first postpartum menstruation. For example, I have a friend who spoke at a New York conference on natural child spacing. She had been in amenorrhea for a long time but realized from her observations that she had ovulated recently and would start her period at the conference. She brought along the necessary equipment, and she did indeed start her first postpartum period at the conference. The mothers in attendance were simply amazed that she knew ahead of time that this would happen. Furthermore, a nursing mother can nurse as long as she desires and still practice natural family planning successfully.

Systematic NFP is easy to learn, easy to use, inexpensive, and healthy. It involves current history. You know on a day-by-day basis if you are fertile or infertile. It can be used to avoid a pregnancy or to achieve a pregnancy. In fact, *The Art of Natural Family Planning* offers a whole chapter of suggestions helpful to those couples having a difficult time achieving a pregnancy.

Some basic physiology

The normal fertility cycle is much better understood than the relationship between nursing and its effect upon fertility. What follows is a simplified version of what happens, and it's not intended to teach you how to practice systematic NFP. However, it will give you a basic understanding of your normal fertility cycle and how that knowledge is used in modern natural family planning.

A few days after your period stops, but sometimes sooner, your brain tells your pituitary gland, a small organ at the base of your brain, to send out a sign that says, "Let's ovulate." That pituitary hormone is called FSH, follicle-stimulating hormone, and it stimulates a follicle in one of your ovaries to begin to develop. (The ovary is your "egg basket," and each egg is contained in an individual follicle.) As the follicle develops, it secretes estrogen, a basic female hormone that has several important effects. The first of these you can't see; it causes the inner lining of the uterus to develop. It has two more effects that you can see or experience. First of all, estrogen causes some cells in the cervix to secrete a mucus discharge which is necessary for normal fertility. (The cervix is the lower end of the uterus that protrudes slightly into the vagina.) This mucus starts out as a rather tacky or sticky substance and then typically becomes like raw egg white. Its function is to aid sperm life and migration. Your mucus discharge is a very positive sign that you are fertile and that the marriage act at this time could cause pregnancy.

Estrogen also causes physical changes in the cervix itself. It tends to rise slightly, the mouth of the cervix opens just a bit, and the tip becomes softer. Most women can notice one or more of these changes if they desire to do so.

You can notice cervical mucus both at the outer lips of the vagina and at the cervix itself. The changes in the cervix are observed by an internal exam. Some women find they get adequate information from the external observation of the cervical mucus; others find the internal mucus observation very helpful.

After about a week of FSH and estrogen activity, ovulation occurs: an egg is released from an ovary and is picked by a fallopian tube to start its journey toward the uterus. If you have relations at the fertile time, sperm and egg can meet in the tube. Their union is called conception or fertilization, and the result is a new human being. If conception occurs, about a week later your newly conceived baby implants in your uterus.

After ovulation, the follicle that released the egg gets a new look and a new name: it becomes yellowish and is called the corpus luteum, Latin for yellow body. The corpus luteum secretes the second basic female hormone, progesterone, and this hormone has several effects on the fertility cycle. First of all, it maintains the inner lining of the uterus and gives it a rich blood supply in preparation for possible implantation. Secondly, it causes your temperature to rise slightly but noticeably. Thirdly, in conjunction with decreased levels of estrogen, it causes the mucus discharge to stop and the cervix changes to reverse — the cervix becomes lower and firmer and the opening closes. Last but not least, progesterone suppresses further ovulations in that cycle.

If pregnancy is not achieved in any given cycle, the corpus luteum stops secreting progesterone—generally about 12 to 16 days after ovulation. The lining of the uterus can no longer be sustained, and it is sloughed off in the process of menstruation. And the cycle begins again.

The bottom line is this: there are three commonly recognized signs of fertility and infertility: mucus, temperature, and cervix. You can learn to observe these. You can use two or three of them in a cross-checking way that is called the sympto-thermal method, or you can use a single-sign system such as mucus-only or temperature-only. This information is helpful in avoiding or achieving pregnancy. It can be used effectively in normal or irregular cycles, and you can use it to monitor the return of fertility while breastfeeding.

Fertility awareness for the nursing mother

Some nursing mothers who experience ovulation prior to menstruation in a lengthy amenorrhea find the cervix sign extremely helpful. Other nursing mothers detect the return of fertility or menstruation by the mucus sign. For example, I did not ovulate prior to my first menstruation, but I knew when menstruation was returning by the mucus sign a few days beforehand.

The temperature sign is also very helpful to the nursing mother. When fertility returns, nursing mothers might notice the more-fertile mucus during the early days of a well-established upward temperature shift. This is common for breastfeeding mothers. Such a mother who is avoiding pregnancy and who is using *only* the mucus sign would have to abstain during this time. The same mother who is using the temperature sign along with the mucus sign can switch to a temperature-only rule (taught by the Couple to Couple League) and the time of abstinence could be shortened.

Even couples desiring pregnancy should chart daily waking temperatures; the temperature shift is the best indicator of the unborn baby's age and can be extremely helpful if any concerns develop later. Oftentimes with nursing, ovulation and the temperature shift may occur one or two weeks later than usual. If this happens and conception occurs, your true due date would be one or two weeks later than an estimate based on your last menstrual period. In addition, you will know when you are pregnant by your chart. With three weeks of elevated temperatures, you have a 99% certainty that you are pregnant. The knowledge attained by charting your fertility signs can be very practical.

The Couple to Couple League

Never before in human history has it been so easy for so many couples to learn their own times of fertility and infertility and to learn natural child spacing through breastfeeding. My husband and I founded the Couple to Couple League in 1971 to spread the knowledge about systematic natural family planning as well as ecological breastfeeding. The Couple to Couple League now has chapters throughout the United States and in 24 foreign countries.

The above general description is not intended to prepare you to use systematic NFP. You would be silly to try to practice any form of systematic NFP or to think you are well prepared to detect your return of postpartum fertility based on the brief description above. Learning natural family planning is like learning to tie your shoes. At first it looks complicated. Then it's so easy once you learn it. To help couples achieve the mastery they need, we have developed both a teaching program with a series of four classes and the *CCL Home Study Course*. The best way to learn the method is to attend the classes taught by a certified Teaching Couple trained by the Couple to Couple League. The *Home Study Course* was developed so that couples who do not live near teachers can learn natural family planning in the privacy of their homes. Both the classes and the *CCL Home Study Course* use *The Art of Natural Family Planning* as a key ingredient.

The Art of Natural Family Planning, the *CCL Home Study Course*, certain books, and many brochures are now available in Spanish from the Couple to Couple League. For continued support and information, the Couple to Couple League publishes a bi-monthly magazine, *CCL Family Foundations*. This magazine continually receives high praise from its readers.

Can you learn to detect the signs of fertility if you're learning this for the first time while pregnant or breastfeeding? Very definitely, yes. Certainly it's easier to learn during the normal cycles, but while you are pregnant or nursing you can learn what to look for and know it later when you experience it. Many women before you have already done it.

Mini-Catalog

The following is a sample of items which are available through the Couple to Couple League catalog. The full catalog contains many items chosen for the support they provide marriages and families and is available upon request. It is also available at the CCL website (www.ccli.org). Current prices are stated in the website and in the current CCL catalog.

Natural Family Planning Materials

The Art of Natural Family Planning by John and Sheila Kippley

The CCL manual explains the sympto-thermal method of natural family planning, as well as mucus-only and temperature-only systems. Completely re-written, revised and expanded in 1996. Large format (8 ½ x 11 inches); easy to read and understand. Also has information on breastfeeding, cycle irregularities, miscarriages, family size, effectiveness, pharmaceutical products and NFP, and much more. Contains a Practical Applications Workbook with answers — for practice in applying the principles and rules.

Daily Observation Charts

A set of 14 charts in a handy booklet form.

Mercury Basal Temperature Thermometer

Modest cost includes shipping.

CCL Family Foundations

This informative support magazine is published six times a year to keep couples up-to-date on systematic natural family planning, ecological breastfeeding, and related family issues.

CCL Home Study Course

The best way to learn NFP without attending classes. Now features the new CCL manual with self-test questions after each chapter. A guide booklet, a CCL membership (this includes the *CCL Family Foundations* magazine), a thermometer, booklet of charts, and brochures and pamphlets, and a review of your first three charts are included in the purchase. If you want more information, request CCL's free descriptive flier.

Birth Control and Christian Discipleship by John F. Kippley

This booklet recalls the pre-1930 universal Christian biblical teaching against unnatural forms of birth control, the Anglican and Protestant departure from that teaching in 1930, and the birth control issue in the light of Christian discipleship.

Fertility, Cycles and Nutrition by Marilyn M. Shannon

This book explains how many cycle irregularities can be either eliminated or alleviated through better nutrition or improved body balance; invaluable to NFP couples and teachers.

Breastfeeding/Parenting

The Womanly Art of Breastfeeding by La Leche League
The best how-to-do-it guide. The standard on breastfeeding.

The American Academy of Pediatrics Policy Statement on Breastfeeding

Excellent 1997 paper showing the current research and the benefits of breastfeeding. Mothers are encouraged to nurse for at least one year, with exclusive breastfeeding the first 6 months. Pediatricians are encouraged to promote, protect, and support breastfeeding.

Medications and Mothers' Milk by Thomas Hale, R. Ph., Ph. D.

An excellent resource written for health professionals. Updated annually. Helps professionals to determine if a medication is safe for nursing mothers and to suggest alternatives.

The Crucial First Three Years by Sheila Kippley

This booklet is Chapter 12 of *Breastfeeding and Natural Child Spacing*. Scientific support for mothers to stay home with their small children.

Nighttime Parenting by William Sears, M.D.

Points out the merits of the family bed and offers advice for problem situations involving sleep.

The Family Bed by Tine Thevenin

Advocates co-sleeping as a way to solve bed and nighttime problems with young children and give them a greater sense of security.

Breastfeeding: Does It Really Space Babies?

Brochure briefly describes the ecological breastfeeding that spaces babies and how to detect the return of fertility. Available in Spanish.

Summary of Mothering-Breastfeeding-Child Spacing Program

A reproducible one-page summary of natural child spacing.

Women's Health

Managing Morning Sickness by Marilyn Shannon

Very helpful booklet that explains what causes morning sickness, what role a woman's diet plays, and what diet and supplements to consider.

Squatting: The Position for Labor and Birth by Megan Steelman, ACCE

A highly recommended brochure. Many vertical positions are illustrated and the benefits listed.

What Your Doctor May Not Tell You About Menopause by John Lee, M.D.

This book is critical of standard hormone replacement therapy with synthetic hormones and instead recommends the use of natural progesterone. Good information about hormones, menopause, and osteoporosis. Written primarily for menopausal women.

What Your Doctor May Not Tell You About Premenopause by John Lee, M.D.

Much of the same content but directed toward women still in their fertile years.

Marriage

Marriage Is for Keeps by John F. Kippley

An excellent guide for preparing couples for Christian marriage with emphasis on the permanence and covenant aspects of marriage.

Informative Videos

Natural Family Planning: Safe, Healthy, Effective by CCL

A video designed for any situation where a brief, biological introduction to systematic NFP is needed, e.g., doctors' offices and marriage preparation. 10 minutes.

Sex Has a Price Tag by Pam Stenzel

One of the best videotapes on this topic. Highly recommended for teenagers and young adults. A strong and clear message for chastity.

Reality Check by Challenge Task Force on Chastity

Many short witnesses to chastity with attractive editing and music. 23 mintues. Comes with a manual.

Informative Audiotapes

"Birth Control! Get the Facts! Know the Truth!" by RADIX

An interview with Dr. Paul Hayes, an OB/GYN who does not prescribe or promote any unnatural forms of birth control. This tape is for teenagers and may be reproduced.

"I Kissed Dating Goodbye" by Josh Harris

Two engaging talks given to teens and parents on how to look at dating in a new light. Maintains that the present dating system is misguided and harmful to young people. Encourages teens to delay dating and instead to focus on finding God's will for this stage of life.

Resource Organizations

For Natural Family Planning Information
The Couple to Couple League
P. O. Box 111184
Cincinnati OH 45211-1184
(513) 471-2000
Charge orders only: (800) 745-8252
Website: www.ccli.org
E-mail: ccli@ccli.org
For materials recommended in this book, please see the mini-catalog at the back of the book.

For NFP-Only Physicians
One More Soul
616 Five Oaks Avenue
Dayton, Ohio 45406
(800) 307-7685
Web Page: www.omsoul.com
Email: omsoul@juno.com

For Breastfeeding Information
La Leche League International
P. O. Box 4079
Schaumburg IL 60168-4079
(847) 519-7730
(800) LALECHE
Web Page: www.lalecheleague.org
E-mail: lllihq@llli.org

Index